K ERRIE H AINS

Exercise Physiologist
Exercise Scientist & Personal Trainer

Back Health
& Core Stability

**Have you ever suffered from back pain?
Do you still suffer from back pain?**

The intention of this book is to teach you the skills to alleviate common causes of back pain and dysfunction. Techniques to release facilitated (tight) muscles, and activate those muscles that are inactive are included in here. It it hoped this book will help improve your posture, function, and prevent recurring pain.

Each exercise is a progression from the one prior, and together they all make up a huge puzzle for you to put together.

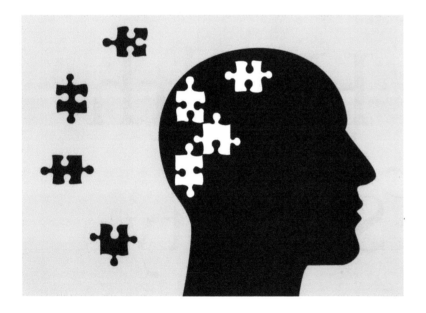

By the end of the book, it is hoped you will be armed with the knowledge of what stretch and exercise you need to do to help prevent, and relieve, your pain on any specific day.

The anatomical diagrams in this book are not drawn to exact origin and insertions. They are designed to give you a general guideline as to where a muscle is, and what action it is designed to perform.

Waiver

Every effort has been made to ensure that the contents of this book are as technically correct, accurate, and sound as possible. The author and the publishers cannot accept responsibility for any injury or loss sustained as a result of the use of this material or the equipment recommended.

There is always a risk in undertaking any physical activity. Your participation in the physical activity recommended in this book is voluntary and done entirely at your own risk.

Consult your health physician before performing any physical activity, particularly if you have an underlying condition.

Ensure that you warm up adequately prior to undertaking any physical activity, or exercise in this book.

Do not perform any exercise incorrectly. Always regress the exercise if your technique is compromised. Gradually work up to performing the more challenging exercises.

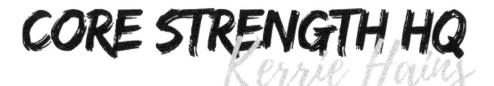

CORESTRENGTHHQ.COM

Welcome to your back health program

I have spent over 30 years working with people, training them for sports performance, general health and fitness, and rehabilitating from injuries and accidents. Over the years, I became very proficient at working on people's back pain and injuries and had a great deal of success with each individual.

As a result of the years of experience I have had, I have put together a number of specific stretches and exercises that have proven time and again, to help people ease and even eliminate their back pain.

This book is designed to give you the knowledge that you need to help yourself prevent, ease, reduce, even eliminate, and be in control of your back pain forever.

Essentially, the book is a progression of stretches and exercises that form a program.

In the program you will learn how to:

Perform specific stretches to release facilitated muscles, and therefore reduce chronic pain.

Alleviate back pain and dysfunction.

Strengthen specific core musculature that directly affect the back and pelvis. Improve posture, function, balance, body awareness, and muscle control. Help prevent further degeneration of your spine.

Improve back health and function. Help prevent injuries in your spine.

Decide what exercise needs to be done on any particular day.

There are a series of stretches and exercises given to you. Each exercise is given in a specific sequence.

Progressing to the next level or exercise is discussed and explained at each point.

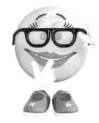

TABLE OF CONTENTS

The Plan

Each activity, stretch, and exercise, is described here in a specific order.

It is recommended you perform the first four activities ('Rotations for Mobility', 'How to Support Your Head', 'Deep Neck Flexor Activation', and 'Pelvic Floor and Transverse Abdominis Activation'), every day for at least one to two weeks, before you move on to the other exercises

It is extremely important to get the very basics of spinal mobility and deep spinal stability correct before moving on to the larger muscle groups that affect your back.

Correct technique for each and every activity in this book is of the utmost importance. If you perform one activity incorrectly and progress to the next one, you increase the risk of further pain and dysfunction.

It is extremely important each activity is performed with correct technique and with the correct muscles activating. Once you know the correct muscles are working, when they are supposed to, with correct muscle firing sequence, and not having other muscles activating to help perform the job, then you can progress to the next activity.

You may find that you need to spend many hours on some activities before you are capable, confident, and able to perform the technique exactly right.

Progress to the next exercise when you have perfected the one you are working on.

Come-in to this program with the intention of doing everything correctly, and learning the techniques properly. This is not a program that you can race through and have no back pain immediately.

However, if you perform every activity correctly, you should notice a reduction in your pain levels.

As you progress through the program, you may find some of the activities are really beneficial for you. You can come back to these at any time and continue to perform them on a regular basis.

It is most important you do every exercise properly before you progress to the next exercise. If you do something wrong you can end up taking three steps backwards, or even more.

You can expect to have some set backs, we don't want poor technique, or rushing through the program to be a cause.

Focus on progressing each step of the way.

Focus on using the right muscles all the time.

Focus on the correct technique all the time.

The exercises shown here are predominately isolation exercises, with a small progression to integrated functional exercises. They are designed to help you activate your core musculature in a safe position.

As you become stronger and more able to activate your core stabilisers, it is expected you will be able to progress to more functional exercises.

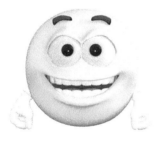

The purpose of this book is to teach specific muscles to stabilise your vertebrae. This is not only for when the trunk is upright, or in a lying down position. It is to teach these muscles to stabilise the trunk against any rotational force and when you are doing your activities of daily life.

Some readers may find that doing certain exercises cause pain. If this is the case, leave that exercise and move to the next one. If you find the next one causes pain as well, regress right back to the beginner four exercises.

At all times listen to your body. Do not do anything that could compromise your back health and core stability.

Some readers may feel more comfortable in flexion rather than extension.

Rotations for Mobility

This first activity is a stretch.

For an exercise to be effective, we must first stretch what is tight, before we strengthen what is weak, or not active.

To do this we need to be very specific about how we stretch, and what we stretch.

Specific gentle stretching is essential.

We have muscles that attach to each joint. These muscles are similar to spokes on a wheel; where the joint is the axel and the spokes are the muscles affecting that joint.

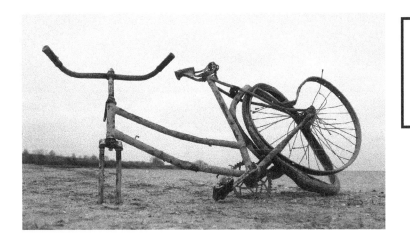

If one of these muscles is tighter than the others, it will directly affect the position of the joint as well as the muscles that attach to that joint.

Typically, when a muscle is facilitated (active or shortened), that is the first muscle to turn on when you try to move that joint. So what happens over time is, that this muscle gets worked more and more. The other muscles around the joint, generally become less active, because they are in a lengthened position.

When a muscle is in a lengthened position, it is more difficult to activate it.

The result is a 'muscle imbalance', some muscles become too tight, and facilitated (always activated), others become too long, and inactive.

All of these muscles are then unable to perform their correct function, and the muscles themselves around the joint break down, and/or, the joint itself gets pulled into a position that is not ideal for fluid movement.

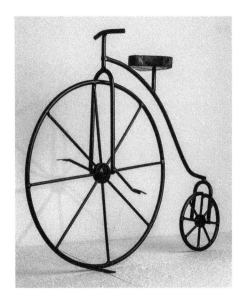

To be effective in our exercise, we must 'turn off', or relax, the facilitated muscles first. The intention of this is to put all the muscles in their correct resting length so they can turn on when they are supposed to, without creating further muscle imbalances.

To turn off facilitated muscles you need to 'tell' your brain it is okay to relax these muscles. To achieve this deactivation of facilitated muscles, you must stretch in a very specific manner and for a specific length of time.

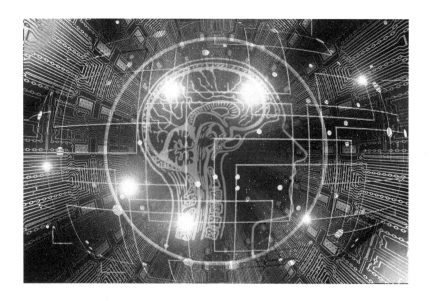

Range of motion stretching must be performed very gently, with minimal load on the spine, and with minimal muscle activation around the vertebrae. To do this, it must be performed lying down with the body totally relaxed.

Instructions:

You should predominately feel this stretch in your lower back area.

Lie on your back, with your feet slightly more than hip width apart. Your legs need to be bent. Your arms need to be out, with your palms up.

Your neck must be neutral. (Ensure you do not have a pony tail in your hair!).

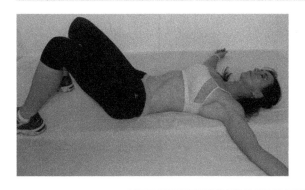

Very slowly, take your legs as far as you feel comfortable to one side. Allow the soles of your feet to come off the floor. Ensure your shoulders stay on the floor and your head stays in neutral.

Do not hold the stretch on any side for more than one full second.

The movement should be very fluid; constant, slow, and controlled.

The constant, gentle, movement will allow the muscles to lengthen as well as relax.

Note: If you do this action too fast, or too slow, you will not gain benefit from the stretch.

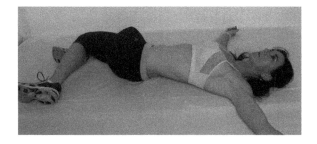

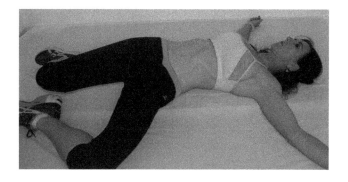

Very slowly move over to the other side, as far as you feel comfortable. Keep your shoulders on the floor.

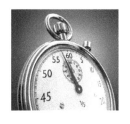

The time taken to perform this stretch is extremely important.

If you perform the range of motion stretch for anything less than one minute, you will not achieve lengthening and relaxing of the muscles.

You need to 'listen' to your body at all times. Once you have performed the stretch consistently for over two minutes, you should notice a point that the tight muscles actually start to relax and 'give'. If it feels like the muscle/s has relaxed as much as it is going to then you can progress to the next step.

If you feel like you could achieve further lengthening and relaxing of the muscle/s, i.e. the muscle/s still feel tight, continue with these rotations for a period of time.

My suggestion for this stretch is to perform the stretch incorporating legs only, keeping your head fixed for at least two to five minutes in total.

Once you have done rotations with only your legs for two to five minutes, then you need to incorporate your head into the stretch. By doing this, you are then affecting further up your spine. At all times, your shoulders should stay on the floor, and you should be continually moving through your full range of motion, to alternate sides.

Turn your head to the opposite side that your legs move to.

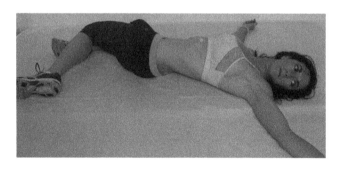

The recommended time frames can be increased if the need be.

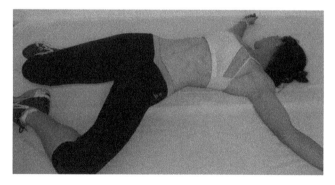

Do not hold the stretch on any side for more than one full second. The movement should be very fluid; constant, slow, and controlled.

The constant, gentle, movement will allow the muscles to lengthen as well as relax.

Note: If you do this action too fast, or too slow, you will not gain benefit from the stretch.

Some people will need to stretch for a lot longer in order to achieve satisfactory muscle relaxation, and lengthening. The most important thing is that you listen to your body and you continue stretching until you notice a change or definite relaxing of the muscle/s.

The more frequently you perform this stretch, you should notice the muscles require less time to attain relaxation and lengthening. If you need to stretch for five minutes with each stretch initially, you may find that over time, you only need two to three minutes to achieve the same effect of muscle relaxation.

What not to do:

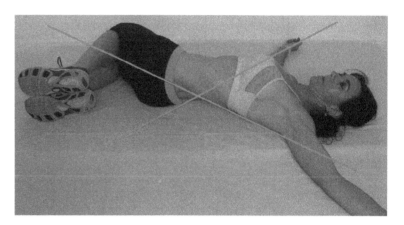

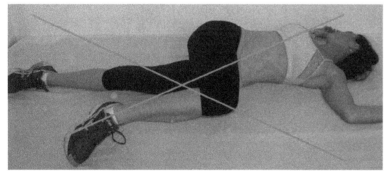

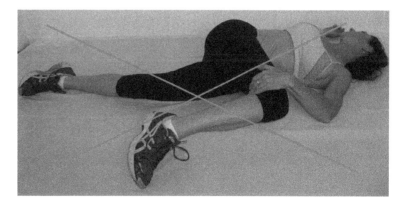

Deep Neck Flexor Activation

A brief look at the anatomy of the neck muscles should help to clarify the need for deep neck flexor muscle activation.

The origin and insertion of a muscle, (where it starts and where it finishes), determine the muscles' action and purpose.

The smaller/shorter a muscle is, the more likely its role is to stabilise.

The larger/longer a muscle is, the more likely its role is to create movement.

There are two muscle groups called the Longus Capitis and Longus Colli muscles. These two muscle groups act as stabilisers for the neck (cervical vertebrae).

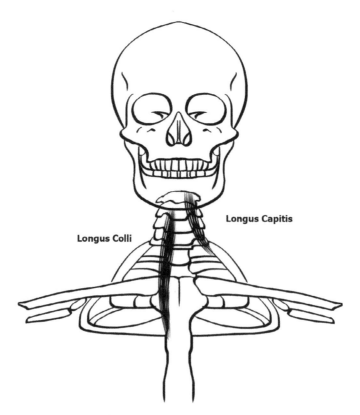

Longus Coli & Longus Capitis Muscles

Diagram 1

We have many other muscles located around the neck and shoulder area that directly affect the head and neck. Some of these include the scalenes and the sternocleidomastoid (SCM) muscles.

If you look at the size and the origins and insertions of these muscles, it should be obvious these two muscle groups are predominately responsible for movement.

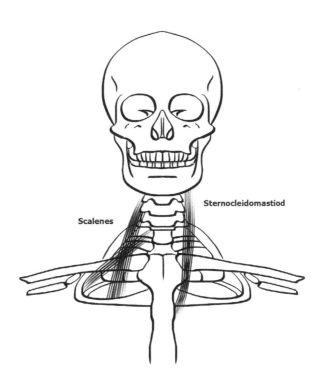

Scalenes and Sternocleidomastoid Muscles

Diagram 2

Typically if the longus colli and longus capitis muscles have 'forgotten' how to turn on due to injury, trauma, or poor posture, these other two muscle groups (scalenes and SCM) will activate and try to do a job they are not good at i.e. stabilise the vertebrae. Invariably, it does not happen well at all. Hence we get neck pain and headaches.

Instructions:

Ensure you have performed the 'Rotations for Mobility' beforehand. This will help relax the SCM and scalenes.

Place a sphygmomanometer (a blood pressure cuff) under your neck. Lie on the floor with your spine neutral.

Pump the sphygmomanometer up to 20mmHG.

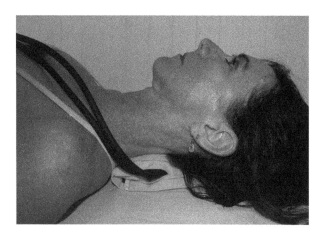

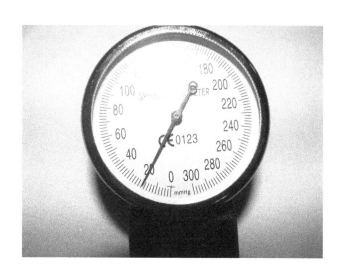

Place your tongue towards the roof of your mouth, your teeth apart, and your lips together.

Give yourself a slight double chin and you should see the needle of the sphygmomanometer move up to 26-28mmHg.

Do not allow the needle to go any higher.

Ensure you have the right muscles activated. If you don't, you will end up giving yourself a headache.

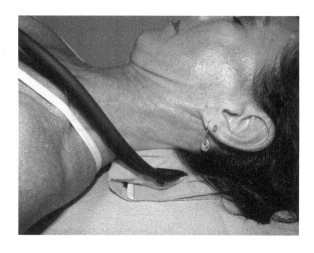

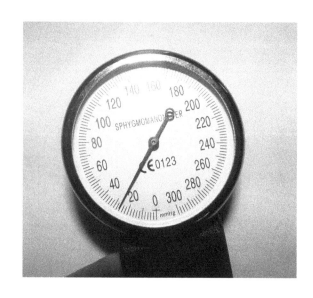

Initially aim to hold this contraction for ten to fifteen seconds to begin with.

Gradually, aim to build up to holding this muscle contraction for 60 seconds.

If you don't have access to a sphygmomanometer, you can use a rolled up hand towel. However, I recommend you do the exercise initially with a sphygmomanometer so you know exactly what you need to do.

The needle is great for biofeedback. Without the needle, you do not know if you are activating too forcefully and therefore potentially causing further muscle imbalances.

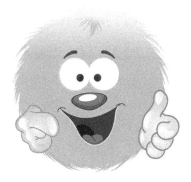

Once you are confident you can activate your deep neck flexors (DNF), then you need to start integrating this muscle contraction into everyday life.

Perform a number of repetitions so you have activated your deep neck flexors for at least three to five minutes in total per session.

Be aware when your head is unsupported, your DNF should be activated.

Pelvic Floor and Transverse Abdominis Activation

Your abdominal muscles are made up of 4 different muscles.

Rectus abdominis
External obliques
Internal obliques
Transverse abdominis

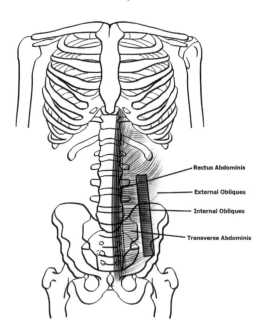

Abdominal Muscles
Diagram 3

The abdominal muscle that is responsible for spinal stability and assists with back strength and function, is the transverse abdominis (TrA).

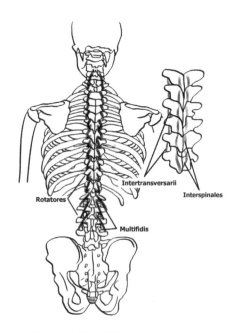

Spinal Stabilisers
Diagram 4

This muscle wraps around from front to back and is 'deep' (underneath), to the other abdominal muscles. It is otherwise known as a 'corset' and performs the role of a corset (i.e. tightens) when activated correctly. When this corset tightens, it pulls on the fascia that it attaches to in your back. This pulling activates the little muscles (multifidis, intertransversarii, interspinales, rotatores), that attach to each vertebra, and subsequently these muscles 'swell'. This swelling stops each vertebra from jamming on each other when we move, and we have what is considered good spinal stability.

This corset has a top and a bottom - the top is the diaphragm and the bottom is the pelvic floor. In order to learn to activate your TrA muscle, it is important you use the diaphragm and pelvic floor muscles correctly.

We must first ensure we are breathing properly. The two muscles responsible for breathing are the diaphragm and the intercostals (see pictures below). When you breathe in, the centre of your diaphragm, which is shaped like a parachute, moves down. As a result of this, your tummy should expand. As you breathe out, the centre of your diaphragm rises, and your tummy should fall. If you breathe deep enough you may also see your chest rise and fall.

Your intercostal muscles are the muscles in between each rib, and they assist with raising the rib cage upon inhalation. Generally, other muscles thought to be involved in breathing are considered accessory muscles, and only some of these will be used with deep inhalation.

If we think about pressure inside our corset, when we breathe in the diaphragm moves downwards, and the pressure increases. As we breathe out, the the diaphragm moves back up and the pressure releases. This breathing out and releasing of the pressure is when it is easiest to activate the pelvic floor.

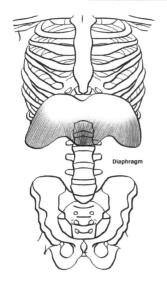

Diaphragm

Diaphragm Muscle
Diagram 5

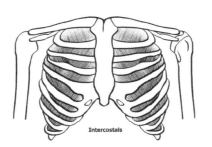

Intercostals

Intercostal Muscles
Diagram 6

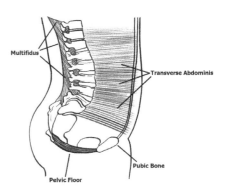

Multifidus

Transverse Abdominis

Pubic Bone

Pelvic Floor

The Pelvic Floor
Diagram 7

Men and women both have pelvic floor muscles and all of us need to exercise these muscles on a regular basis. The pelvic floor muscle is similar to a sling at the base of your corset.

The cue for a female to activate her pelvic floor is: 'pretend you are stopping the flow of urine'. Note: do not practice stopping the flow of urine mid-flow, as this is not recommended at all and may end up confusing your neuromuscular system.

The cue for a male to activate his pelvic floor is: 'pretend you are walking into freezing cold water and you do not want your little boys to touch that water'.

The cues I give when instructing someone to activate their pelvic floor and TrA are as follows:

Lie down on your back with your spine neutral.

Breathe in; your tummy and chest should rise (as a result of air filling the cavity only).

Breathe out; your tummy and chest should fall.

Activate your pelvic floor, as recommended above.

Draw your belly button in.

You should not be able to see anything move except your abdominal wall. Hold this for two to five seconds. Repeat for three minutes.

To ensure that you are activating your TrA correctly, without the use of an ultrasound machine, simply find the top of your pelvic bone, move two centimetres in and two centimetres down. Palpate here: sometimes this needs to be quite deep, depending on the level of subcutaneous fat you have.

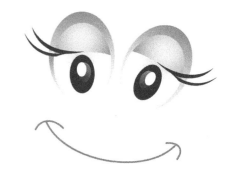

When you activate your pelvic floor and draw your belly button in, you should feel this go hard. It is also recommended that you actively turn this muscle off and feel the muscle soften under your fingers.

If you contract too forcefully, you will feel the muscle go hard, then you will feel your fingers lifting up. This lifting up is your obliques and is not what we want to do. Ease off the intensity and focus on feeling the muscle go hard only.

Just like other muscle slings in the body, the TrA also have slings that work together.

The TrA muscle is 'sectioned' into six 'areas'. Left and right sides and these each have upper, middle and lower areas. These different areas will contract more so than others depending on the action you are performing.

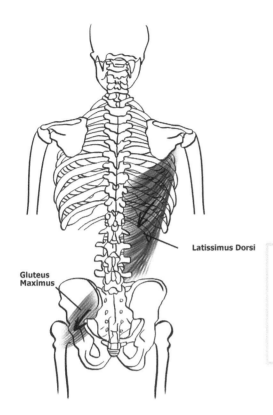

Gluteus
Maximus

Latissimus Dorsi

Muscle Fibre Alignment - showing a muscle sling in the back of the body.
Diagram 8

It is believed that our abdominals are designed to stop motion not create it. They are also designed to transfer power and movement through the trunk. Keeping this in mind, the abdominals should be trained specifically for their function.

Every individual has a history of movement patterns, a history of injuries, and their own current areas of pain. These will affect and influence the effectiveness of a muscle activating. There are many factors that affect the activation and performance of the TrA. These factors include pain, injury, posture, ingrained motor patterns, and body awareness.

If for example you have an injury and therefore pain in your right leg, you tend to limp, or compensate by walking and moving differently. The muscles affected try not to activate due to increased pain. Other muscles then have to turn on to help achieve the task at hand. This can then result in poor motor patterns. You will then find other areas of that leg or hip become quite sore, due to increased demands on them as well as them having to do a job they are not specifically designed to do.

Our bodies are amazing machines. If you want to do something, for example a push up, your body will do the push up, but it may not be using the right muscles and it may not be with the correct posture. This is where injuries result.

Considering 80% of the population will experience back pain in their lives, it can be assumed the majority of readers have this type of issue occurring in their trunks.

Putting it all together:

The TrA have areas of the muscle that will activate more so depending on the demand placed on the body. The trunk has areas where the muscle has become inactive due to pain and dysfunction.

Teaching the TrA to turn on is critical to ensure back health and core stability.

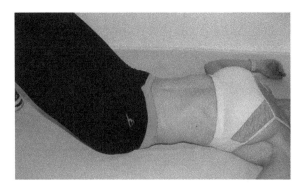

Supine Lying Neutral

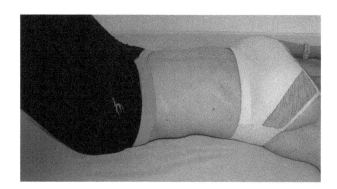

Supine Lying Breathe In

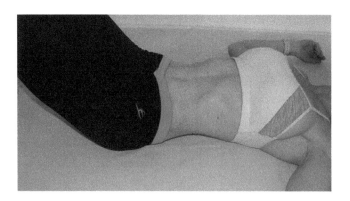

Supine Lying Breathe Out and Activate TrA

Generally most people will teach activation in a supine lying position first then progress them to unsupported positions.

I believe we need to find the supported position that is most effective for each individual to effectively activate their TrA from, then move to the other supported positions.

There are generally four supported positions we can start TrA activation from.

Supine

Side Lying Left

Side Lying Right

Prone

Breathe In	TrA Activation

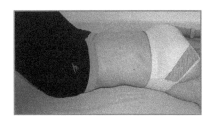 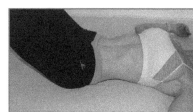 Supine

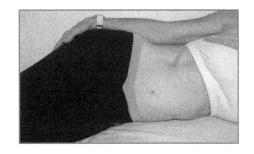 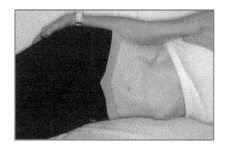 Side Lying Left

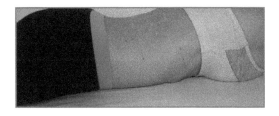 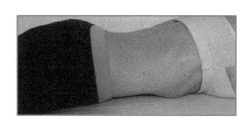 Prone Lying

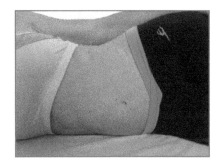 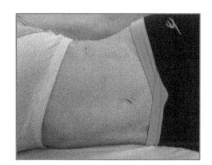 Side Lying Right

When you are starting out, try each position and determine which one is the most effective and 'easiest' for you to activate your core muscles. There is usually one position that is easier than the others.

Work out the next easiest, through to the most difficult position. You should have a list of four positions going from easiest to activate, to the most difficult to activate.

I want you to start with the position that is easiest. Perform your core activation in this position for a total of three minutes. Then move to the next position for three minutes, then the next for three minutes, then the last position for three minutes.

If any of these positions cause you pain or discomfort, you may need to adjust yourself, so you are not in pain. A pillow strategically placed may help you. Remember that your body will avoid pain at all costs and will do the job no matter what. Make sure it is the right job.

Every time you are performing the exercise, your brain and muscles (neuromuscular system) are communicating. Hopefully by the time you have moved to the last position (which is your least easy position), your brain will have some idea of what it is required to do. This will help reinforce correct muscle firing for each position.

Remember, we are training a muscle activation pattern and we want the correct muscles and the correct sequence of muscles to fire at the right time.

This initial phase may take a while to get through, but it is essential you master it before you move on to the next exercises.

As the communication in your neuromuscular system improves, you should notice each position is as easy to activate as each other. This indicates that your brain has formed a connection with the muscles.

Throughout the day, try to be aware of activating your core musculature, and turn the muscles on when you are in sitting, standing, walking, moving... If you notice you are regressing to poor motor patterns, stop. Go back to the supported position and continue here for a few more days.

Once you have mastered the activation lying down in all four positions, you are able to progress to the next exercise in the book.

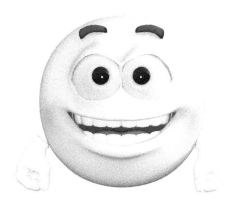

How to Support your Head

The intention of this activity is to teach you how to support your head correctly until such time as your deep neck flexors can do their job properly.

Any time your head is off the floor your deep neck flexors should be active to stabilise your cervical (neck) vertebrae. There are also a number of other muscles around the neck that need to activate. If they don't all work together as they should, the risk of neck pain, dysfunction, and injury increases.

What happens in one part of the spine directly affects every other area of the spine. So correct head positioning, and muscle activation, is essential in the head and neck area.

Correct support of the head is essential to learn before undertaking any exercise that involves your head being unsupported.

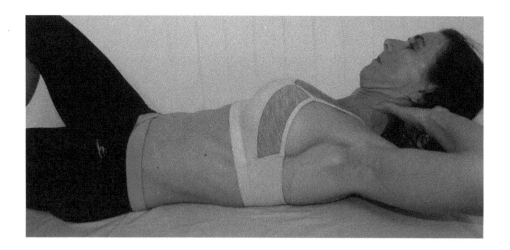

In an ideal world each one of us has deep neck flexors strong enough to support our own head, when we are in any position. Using your hands to correctly support your head is an interim activity that you aim to eventually eliminate.

Instructions:

Place your fingers on your neck. Place your little fingers on the base of your skull. Your thumbs will rest towards the front of your throat.

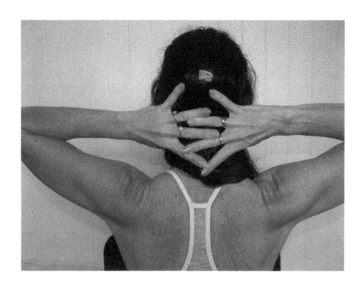

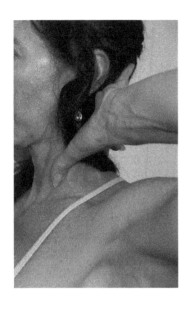

Your little fingers are responsible for holding the weight of your head. The remainder of your fingers are on your neck itself, and this also helps to hold the weight of your head, but prevents you being able to bring your head forward as you lift.

Keep your elbows out to the side. If you bring your elbows in front of you, it tends to encourage you to pull your head forward.

Activate your deep neck flexors as described previously, then slowly lift your shoulders off the floor as if you are a fixed unit from the rib cage up.

Hold for one to two seconds and return back to resting. Repeat for up to ten repetitions.

What not to do:

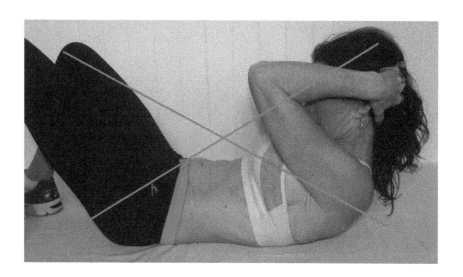

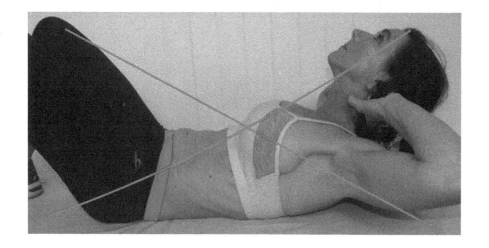

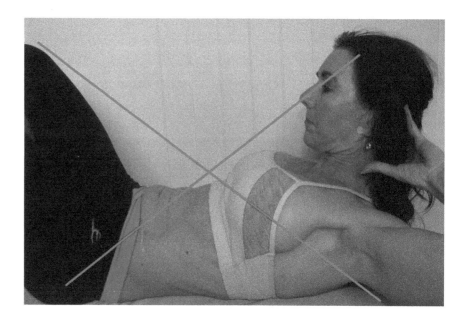

Cat/Cow Stretch

The intention of this stretch is to mobilise your spine in a flexion/extension manner, without creating too much range.

If you are working outside your ideal range with your spine, the risk of pain and dysfunction is much higher.

It is believed that if you are 'too flexible' then you can actually cause more damage and pain to your spine. There is an ideal range of motion for each of us with our spines. We need to find what that range is, and maintain it.

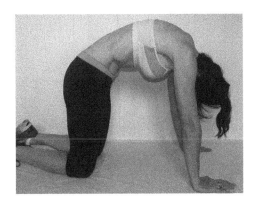

It is imperative you perform this stretch correctly.

We have previously mobilised our spine in a rotation movement, this time we want to mobilise our spine in a flexion/ extension movement (forwards and backwards movement).

If you have any discogenic back pain, you may find your range in this exercise is restricted.

The use of your breath and the activation of specific muscles with this activity will make it more effective.

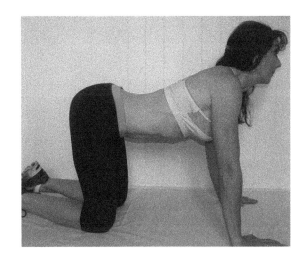

Instructions:

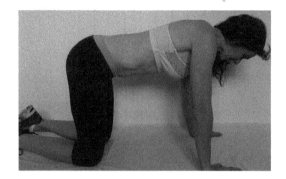

Kneel on your hands and knees. Your hands should be directly under your shoulders. Your knees should be directly under your hips.

Ensure your spine is neutral. Gently move into 'cat' position.

Take a deep breath in. Breathe out. Activate your TrA. Follow through with the activation of these muscles by drawing your tummy in and up. Continue with the activation by arching your back up and encouraging your head and tail bone to lower towards the floor.

Try to encourage the arch of your back by imagining you are making a circle with your spine; your head and tail bone would make the circle complete by joining together.

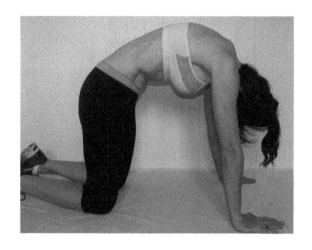

Once you have reached your comfortable full range of motion, you then need to reverse the action. Gently move into 'cow' position.

Slowly breathe out, and as you do tilt your pelvis
so your tail bone lifts as high up towards the sky as
you can. At the same time, extend through the upper
back by encouraging the chest to lower to the floor.

The action is that of extending
(lengthening) your spine, so do not allow
it to collapse.

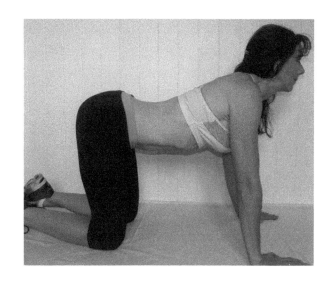

Do not extend your neck backwards.

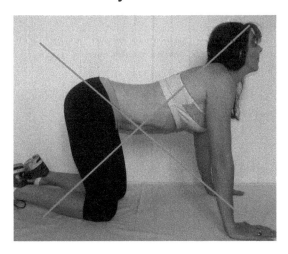

Keep your hip and shoulder joints fixed
and stable. Do not allow them to drop out
of ideal position.

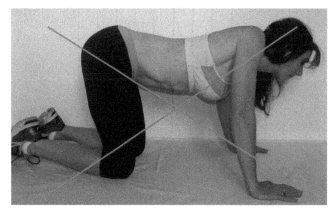

Once you have reached your comfortable end of range, return back to the cat position of the exercise.

Work through your maximum range of motion. Keep in mind, we each have our own specific range.

Continue moving through both cat and cow positions for at least two minutes.

Your speed of movement should be slow, purposeful, and controlled; in time with your breathing.

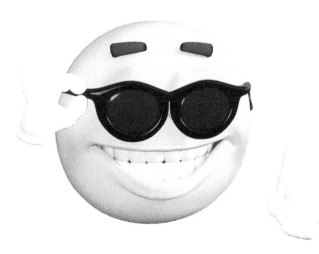

Supine Alternate Leg Lift (Bent Leg)

This exercise is the first progression from 'Pelvic Floor and Transverse Abdominis Activation'.

The intention of this exercise is to teach these muscles to stabilise your pelvis and also stabilise your vertebrae while you move your legs.

If you watch a trained olympic sprinter running down the track towards you, their limbs are moving, while their entire core is totally fixed.

There is a lot of drive and force going through their core, but their core remains totally fixed. Nothing else moves except their limbs.

Our abdominals are designed to transfer force and stop motion.

A highly trained athlete that has correctly functioning transverse abdominis muscles, will be able to sprint down the track, with only their limbs moving.

This is how were are supposed to move at all times. When we walk, run, swim, ride a bike...

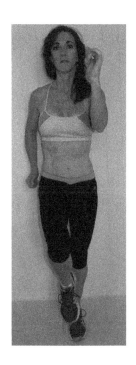 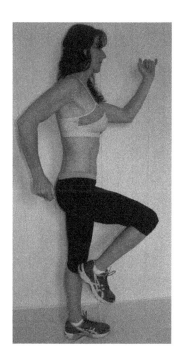

Imagine our bodies are like a car and our trunk is the vehicle itself. Our shoulder and hip joints are our 'axels'. These axels need to be totally fixed and stable in order to have the wheels move in a fluid, correct pattern.

If these 'axels' move around when the wheel (our limbs) are in motion, wear and tear becomes apparent and the joint itself wears out.

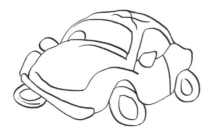

Our joints can potentially wear out.

The same applies to the human body. If our shoulder and hip joints are stable when we move, they move from an ideal point. If our trunk, or body, is not strong enough to hold us in the correct position, then our joints will not move from an ideal position.

If our transverse abdominis do not keep our trunk fixed, we develop pivot points in our vertebrae that cause movement in our trunk. These pivot points potentially become extremely sore, wear out, and stiffen up.

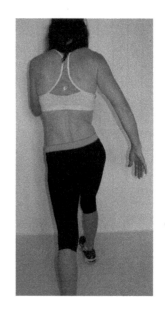

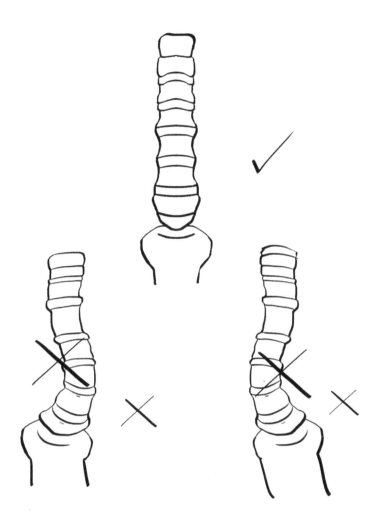

Rotation/Tilting of Pelvis Affecting the Vertebrae

Diagram 9

The role of the TrA is to stabilise our spine in conjunction with the mutlifidis and the pelvic floor. This exercise is designed to teach these muscles to stabilise the pelvis from where they are, i.e. the core.

Instructions:

Ensure you are executing the 'Pelvic Floor and Transverse Abdominis Activation' exercise correctly before you move to this exercise.

Set yourself up the same way as you would for the exercise 'Pelvic Floor and Transverse Abdominis Activation'.

Ensure you keep your spine neutral. Do not arch your back.

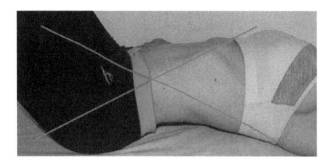

Lie on your back. This places your body in a 'quiet' position, i.e. your body is not under any significant load. Your spine should be totally supported by the floor. Your legs should be bent, with your feet hip width apart.

Place your fingers on your pelvic bones. Breathe in, breathe out, activate your pelvic floor and activate your TrA. Then, lift one leg off the floor.

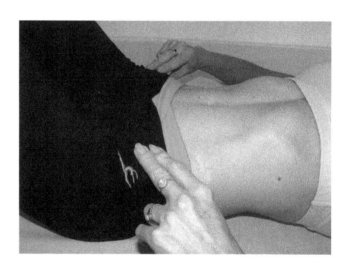

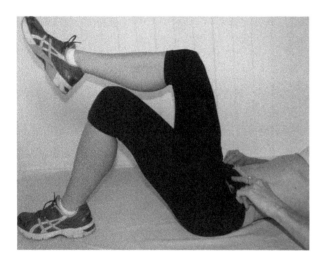

The angle at your knee should stay fixed, you are simply moving from the hip joint.

Relax, breathe in, breathe out, activate your pelvic floor, draw your belly button in, and lift the other leg off the floor and slowly lower it down.

Lower this leg back down so your foot returns to the floor.

The challenge is to keep your pelvis fixed at all times. It should not move, tilt, or twist, at all.

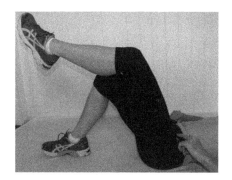

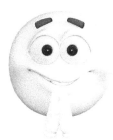

The 'relax and activate core musculature' in between each leg lift, is the first progression. It allows you to rest and reset, if you need to between leg lifts.

Perform this exercise until you are able to keep your pelvis fixed throughout the entire movement.

Note: As soon as you feel the pelvis tilt, or twist, or drop, stop the movement of the leg. Keep the leg fixed. Move the pelvis to where it should be, then continue with lifting the leg.

By doing this you are teaching your neuromuscular system a new movement pattern. It must be repeated a number of times before this becomes a natural motor engram.

When performing the exercise, as soon as you notice you are doing something incorrect, stop, relax, then try it again. This may be made up of one ten-second repetition or the total length of time that you can perform the action correctly. Aim to build up to three minutes continuous.

This exercise should be performed as many times properly as you can for up to three minutes continuously. If you notice you are fatiguing and doing the action wrong, you must stop the exercise.

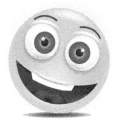

If you can perform the exercise correctly and continuously for three minutes at a time, then you are able to progress to the next exercise.

Once you can perform 'Supine Alternate Leg Lift (Bent Leg)' properly with a reset of the core musculature in between lifting legs, then you can progress to performing the same action without resetting in between each leg lift. This is detailed now.

Breathe in, breathe out, activate your pelvic floor, draw your belly button in. Lift one leg off the floor and slowly lower it down. Keep the contraction of the core musculature, lift the other leg and lower it down.

Once you have returned the second foot to the floor, you can then relax, reset and repeat the exercise.

Again, the pelvis should not move at all throughout the movement.

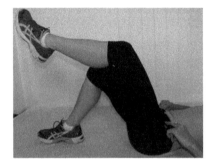

Continue with this purposeful relax, reset, repeat, until you can lift each leg and change legs without the pelvis moving.

Some people may find they need to stop, relax, and consciously activate their core musculature before lifting their other leg. If you are one of these people, take your time until you have mastered this exercise. It is imperative you perform this exercise correctly. Regress if you need to.

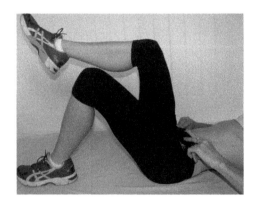

Your next progression is to breathe in, breathe out, activate your pelvic floor, draw your belly button in. Lift one leg off the floor and slowly lower it down, lift the other leg off the floor, slowly lower it down. Continue with lifting and lowering while at the same time you are able to breathe and ensure activation of your core musculature.

These are simple progressions, but imperative they are followed step by step. Advance only when you have mastered the previous exercise.

Your leg is a weight. The longer your leg, the heavier the load. This is why we start with the knee bent and fixed at an angle.

As you become more proficient at the exercise, you can gradually increase the length of your leg, i.e. increase the angle the knee is bent at.

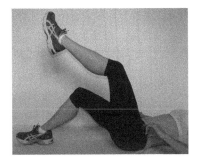 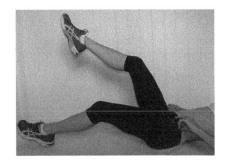

What not to do:

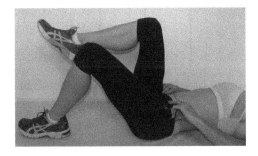 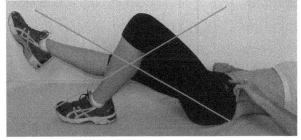

Supine Alternate Leg Lift (Straight Leg)

This is a progression from 'Supine Alternate Leg Lift (Bent Leg)'. Once you can perform that correctly, try this.

Set yourself up the same way as you would for the exercise 'Pelvic Floor and Transverse Abdominins Activation'.

Lie on your back. This places your body in a 'quiet' position. i.e. your body is not under any significant load. Your spine should be totally supported by the floor. Your legs should be almost straight, with your feet hip width apart.

Place your fingers on your pelvic bones. Breathe in, breathe out, activate your pelvic floor, draw your belly button in. Lift one leg off the floor. Lower it slowly to the floor. Lift the other leg off the floor and lower it slowly to the floor.

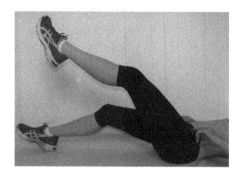 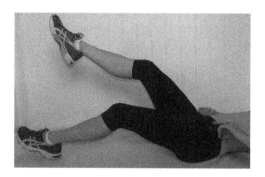

The angle at the knee stays fixed at all times.

The neuromuscular system is learning that when you move your legs this way, your core musculature needs to keep your pelvis and spine fixed.

The intention is that this then translates to every day activities.

Your legs are mimicking the walking action, and we are now training a motor pattern as well as core and pelvic stability.

I encourage people with back pain to be active but if they are out pounding the pavement everyday without being able to stabilise their pelvis and spine, then they could very well be making their back pain worse.

Sometimes it is better to cease the 'walking for fitness' or the 'daily jog' until such time as your body is able to stabilise itself.

It really doesn't take too long to master the exercises. You need to be mindful of what you are doing while you are exercising. You also need to try to avoid any activities that encourage the poor motor patterns.

Each time you perform a poor motor pattern, it reinforces this pattern again. We are trying to create a new motor pattern, so total avoidance of the old motor pattern is desired.

Obliques for Rotation

As part of good core strength and back health we need to teach our obliques what they need to do. Their job primarily is to rotate the trunk, to prevent over rotation, and to assist with supporting the trunk when there is load on it, for example in a push-up position.

When you are in a push up position, ideally your transverse abdominis will activate to stabilise your vertebrae, in conjunction with your spinal stabilisers. Your obliques, both internal and external, will activate together with rectus abdominis, and this stops the 'sagging' we often see in trunks when they are in a bridge position.

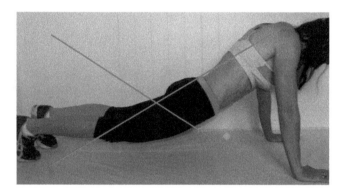

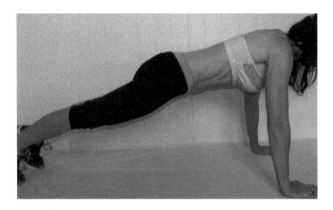

This exercise is designed to teach the obliques to rotate.

Note: the direction of the muscle fibres. The right external obliques work directly with the left internal obliques to cause rotation to the left. The left external obliques work with the right internal obliques to cause rotation to the right. These muscles also work together to prevent over rotation with activities such as walking.

Internal and External Obliques Showing Muscle Fibre Direction
Diagram 10

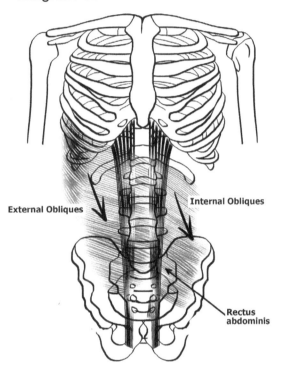

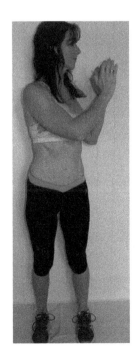 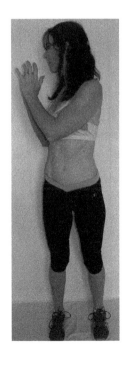

Instructions:

Lie on your back with your spine neutral. Your legs should be bent, with your feet together. Your arms should be out to the sides, with your palms up.

Keep your trunk fixed. Slowly take both legs over to one side. Allow the soles of both feet to come off the floor.

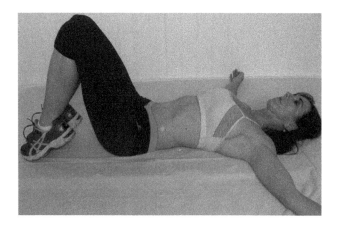

The range your legs attain will be determined by your mobility in your trunk.

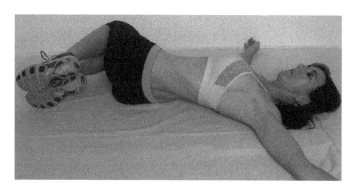

To return your legs to the start position, you need to activate your pelvic floor and transverse abdominis, then, consciously activate your obliques on the opposite side your legs are. Use your obliques to pull your pelvis and therefore, your legs, back to the start position.

Both shoulders must stay on the floor.

As soon as you notice your opposing shoulder lifting off the floor, you must stop your rotation.

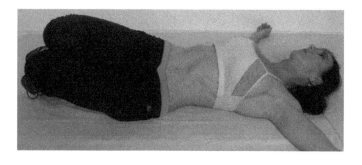

Take your legs to the other side.

Rotate as far as you feel comfortable. Keep both shoulders on the floor. Activate your core musculature. Focus on using your obliques to bring your pelvis and legs back to the centre.

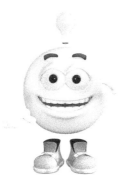

Perform the exercise slow and controlled. Ensure you are using the correct muscles.

If you are doing this exercise properly, you will find that you will stay in the same spot on your mat. If you are using the wrong muscles, you will find that you move down the mat.

To progress the exercise, bend your arms up. This reduces your base of support. Be aware of how much force you are putting on your arms each time you return your pelvis to neutral.

Are you pushing down with your arms to help you?

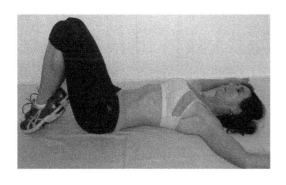
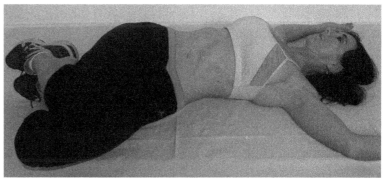

You can progress to the next step if: you have correct muscle activation, you feel your obliques are working, and you are not pushing down on your arms to bring your legs back to the centre.

Note: You can progress even if you cannot get your legs all the way down to the floor.

Lie on your back with your spine neutral. Your legs should be bent, with your feet together. Your arms should be pointing to the ceiling with your palms together.

Keep your trunk fixed. Slowly take both legs over to one side. Allow the soles of both feet to come off the floor.

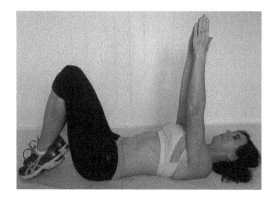

Your hands and arms should remain in line with your sternum, and stay fixed. Your shoulders should stay on the floor.

Lift your heels off the floor and keep your toes on the floor.

Slowly rotate your legs as far as you can to one side. Activate your pelvic floor and transverse abdominis. Then consciously activate your obliques on the opposite side that your legs are. Use your obliques to pull your pelvis and therefore, your legs, back to the start position.

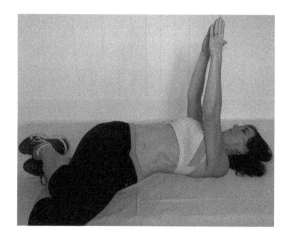

You should notice this exercise is more difficult because you have eliminated your base of support by lifting your arms off the floor.

If you are doing this exercise properly, you will find that you stay in the same spot on your mat. If you are using the wrong muscles, you will find that you move down the mat as the repetitions increase.

You may find one side is more difficult to do the exercise on than the other. This is pretty normal. Work to achieve balance with both sides.

As you work through the exercise session, you may find your range improves and your function improves. This is the intention. You should also notice your pain reduces.

Consciously think all the time when performing the exercise. 'What muscles am I working?' 'What muscles am I supposed to be working?' 'What action am I trying to achieve?'

Your aim is to perform the exercise for three to five minutes at a time. This is dependent on your technique. If you cannot perform the exercise correctly, you must stop the exercise.

Technique is always your guiding factor.

Supine Hip Extension/Prone Hip Extension

This exercise is designed to teach your gluteals to activate. Many times we experience back pain because our gluteals don't do their job properly and our back muscles tend to try to do the job instead.

When a muscle, or muscle group, do a job that they are not designed to, it eventually results in pain, dysfunction and potentially, injury.

The primary function of the gluteus maximus muscle (gluteals) is to extend the hip.

When performing this exercise, correct technique is extremely important.

This exercise is not to be confused with the previous exercises for core musculature activation. This is an exercise in itself. It is designed to teach the gluteals to turn on when you have activated your spinal stabilisers.

To help turn off the back muscles and encourage the gluteals to activate, you need to place the back muscles in a lengthened position. Remember, it is very difficult to turn a muscle on when it is in a lengthened position.

Instructions:

Supine Hip Extension

Lie on your back. Your spine and pelvis should both be neutral. Your legs should be bent, with your feet hip width apart.

Activate your pelvic floor and transverse abdominis. Tilt your pelvis backward. (Imagine there is a bowl of water in your pelvis and you are tipping it out on the floor).

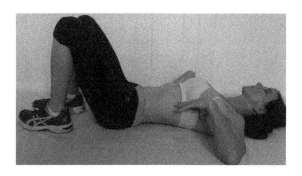

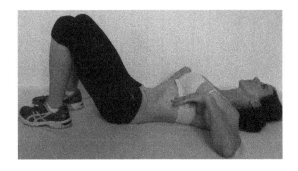

This tilting backward of your pelvis places your back muscles on stretch. This then makes it hard for them to turn on.

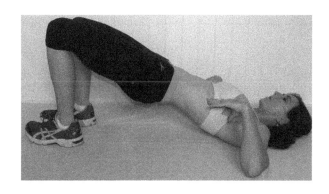

Some of you may not like placing your back in this position. If this is the case, try the 'Prone Hip Extension' instead.

Keep your core musculature activated, consciously activate your gluteals, and try to lift your pelvis off the floor one vertebra at a time.

You may find your hamstrings (muscles at the back of your thigh), cramp. If this is the case, simply lift your toes off the floor.

Ensure your gluteals are on. You may feel your lower back muscles are active, but hopefully they are not primarily responsible for the lifting of the hips. Feel both muscle groups; the gluteals and the lower back muscles. The easiest way to tell if a muscle is on is to feel it. If it feels like the muscle has gone hard, then generally it is active.

Lift up until your knees, hips and shoulders form a straight line, or before your back arches (goes into extension), whichever you reach first. Then slowly lower back down one vertebra at a time.

Knees, hips, and shoulders should form a straight line

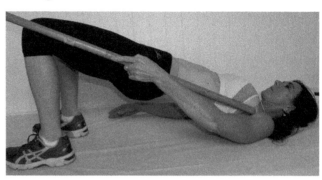

Repeat the exercise for up to ten repetitions, as long as your technique is correct.

Return back to neutral spine. Consciously activate your core musculature, tilt your pelvis backwards, activate your gluteals, and lift your pelvis off the floor one vertebra at a time. Lift to straight. Slowly lower down one vertebra at a time, back to neutral.

The lifting and lowering of the pelvis one vertebra at a time is essential to the success of this exercise. If you do not 'peel' on and off the floor with your back, you will generally be simply lifting straight up, and this allows the back muscles to do the job. Doing this you may be potentially creating more pain and dysfunction.

Palpate your muscles (touch them) throughout the entire movement, so you are aware of how much each muscle is activating.

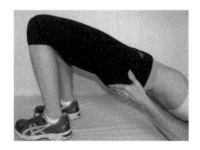 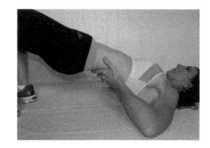

Initially you may find your range to tilt your pelvis is restricted. This is to be expected, especially if you have back pain. Work within your pain range. As you progress through the exercises and the book, you should find your range improves, along with a reduction in your pain levels.

Note: Do not extend up so far that your back goes into extension, or arching. This will jam your discs and potentially cause pain, dysfunction, and injury.

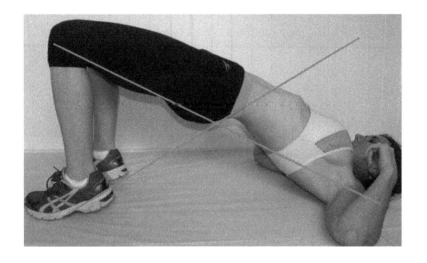

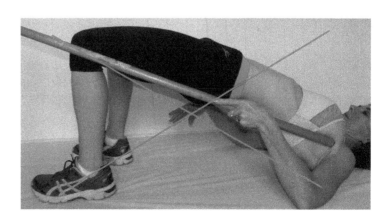

Instructions:

Prone Hip Extension

Lie on your stomach, over a ball. Place your hands on the floor, with your feet touching the floor.

Most of your weight should be on your hands. You spine should be relaxed and your neck should be neutral.

Activate your core musculature and the gluteals of one of your legs. Keep your spine fixed and lift that foot off the floor. You should notice the thigh of that leg lifts off the ball.

Lift the leg up, until the thigh is horizontal. Slowly lower that leg. Repeat the action with the other leg.

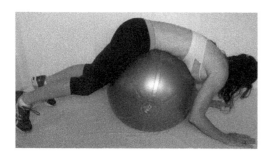

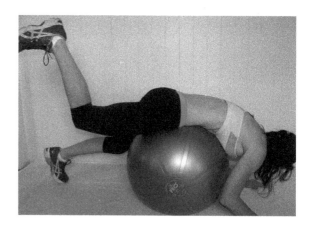

Be aware when doing this exercise, that the pelvis does not rotate, that the spine does not tilt, and that the neck stays neutral.

Concentrate on the activation of the gluteals with every repetition. Palpate (feel) them if you need to. This helps to reinforce to you they are activating.

Palpate (feel) your lower back and ensure it is not activated. There will be a level of muscle activation in your lower back, to help resist the trunk from rotating. This is fine. However, you do not want your lower back to be doing the lifting of the leg, so ensure your gluteals are on and the lower back is only slightly on.

Perform up to fifteen repetitions per leg, as long as they are executed correctly, then change legs. Remember technique determines repetitions.

What not to do:

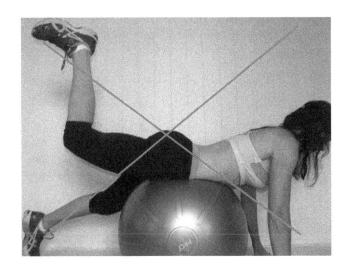

The more relaxed you can make your lower back muscles while you are doing this exercise, the more effective it will be. You do not want to lift your trunk up to horizontal with this exercise.

This exercise can be done on the floor, but it is very difficult to prevent the lower back from activating. If you do not have an exercise ball to perform the exercise on, try placing a cushion under your trunk to help create the relaxed/lengthened position of the lower back muscles.

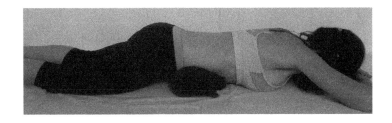

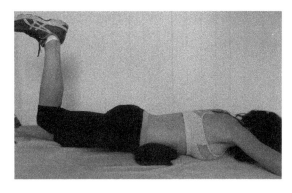

47

Thoracic Stretch

This is a lovely stretch for your back. A lot of people have stiff, sore backs and necks because their thoracic spine is tight.

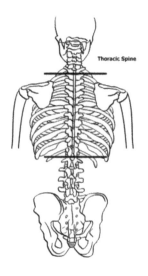

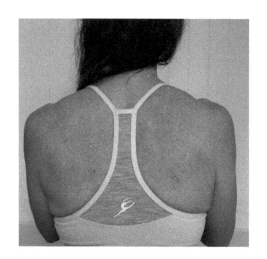

Diagram 11

Generally, what happens in one part of the spine, directly affects all other parts of the spine. So, if you are tight in your thoracic spine, other areas of your back may need to move more freely to maintain the total range of motion your body requires.

Over time, this extra range in other areas of your back cause pain, dysfunction, and then, stiffness in these areas. Then your entire back may become more stiff and more painful.

The intention with this is to gently mobilise your thoracic spine, to take the pressure off other areas of your spine.

Instructions:

Towel Roll

Use a bath towel and fold it length ways so the width of it is about the same width as your body. Then fold it in half. Roll the towel tightly so it will provide a resistance when you lay on it.

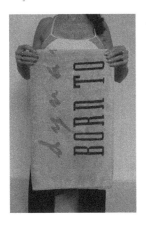 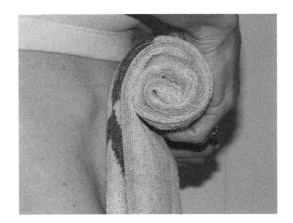

The amount of roll you have with the towel will directly affect the amount of stretch you achieve. Make sure you roll it enough to create a change in your spine.

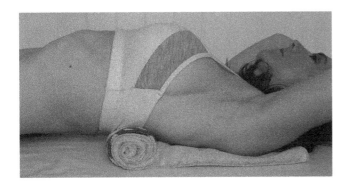 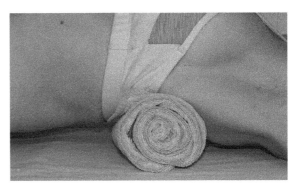

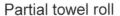

Partial towel roll   Full towel roll

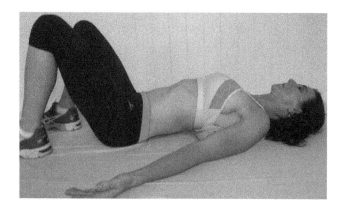 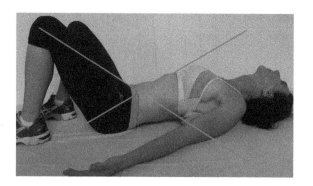

Ensure your neck is elongated

Place the rolled up towel on the floor and lie down on the towel. It should be on your back, directly under your chest.

Try to elongate your neck (do not allow your neck to tip backwards), this will increase the stretch in your thoracic spine.

If you have a level of kyphosis or you are quite thick through the chest area, you may need to place a pillow under your head to support it. Try to ensure that you are still achieving a stretch in your thoracic area.

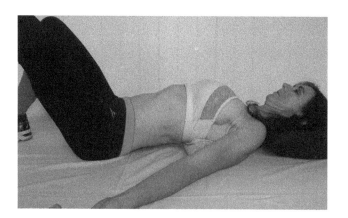

If you can, lie on the towel for up to five to ten minutes at any one time. If you find it uncomfortable, reduce the amount of stretch by reducing the size of the roll in the towel, but try to maintain the length of time you perform the stretch.

Ensure that your palms are up, that your neck is elongated, and that your legs are bent. Focus on relaxing through the thoracic spine every time you breathe out.

You may find when you have finished the stretch, that you are unable to sit straight up. If this is the case, simply roll to the side, off the towel.

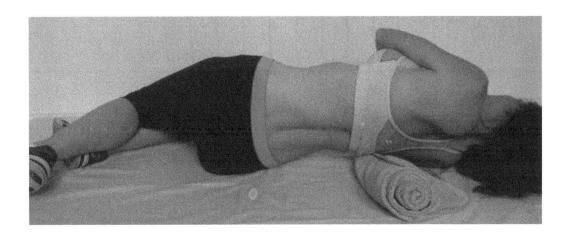

As you become more mobile in your thoracic spine, you should be able to increase the thickness of the towel roll.

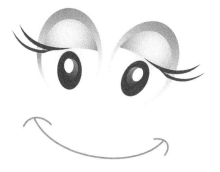

Instructions:

Thoracic Stretch Using Arms

If you don't have any shoulder issues and you are able to put your shoulders in the position shown, then try the following stretch.

Kneel on the floor. Bend your arms and place the backs of your arms on the ball as shown.

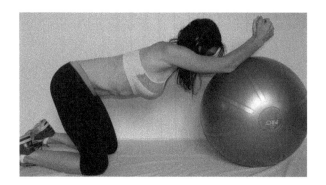 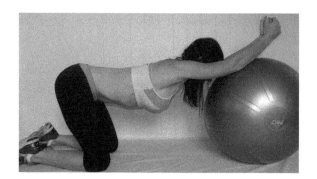

Keep your neck neutral, and try to push your chest and thoracic spine down. Ensure you are not arching your back.

Hold the stretch for six to eight seconds, relax and repeat four to five times.

What not to do:

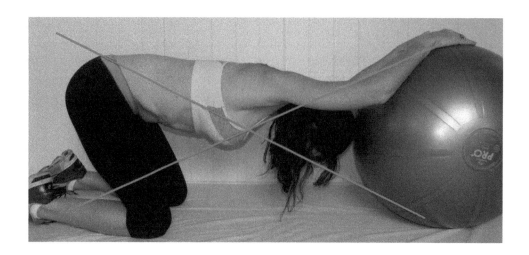

Scapula Control

The intention of this exercise is to teach the muscles around our shoulder blades (scapulae) their correct job.

If you look at the shoulder blade (scapula) itself, it is basically a triangular shape. Muscles attach to the scapula from all directions.

It is very common to have these muscles become unbalanced in their length and their strength. It is ideal to have equal length tension in all of these muscles to ensure the scapula sit in their correct place and move and function correctly.

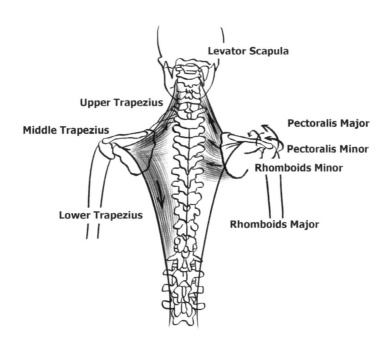

Muscles Directly Affecting the Shoulder Blade
Diagram 12

If we have muscle imbalances around the shoulder girdle and scapula area, generally it is because the chest muscles are shorter, tighter and/or stronger than the opposing muscles in the back area. Another contributing factor is that the muscles that attach to the upper portion of the scapula tend to get worked more than the muscles that attach to the lower potion of the scapula.

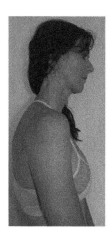

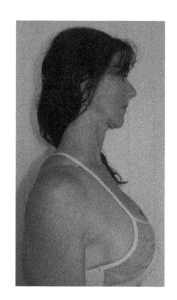

Poor posture showing internal
rotation of the shoulders.

Ideal positioning of the shoulders

As previously stated, in order to achieve correct muscle
balance we need to stretch what is tight, before we
strengthen what is weak. This stretching itself should also
help to put your shoulder joint in a more favourable position.

**Generally, it is the mid and lower
trapezius, and rhomboid major
muscles that need strengthening.**

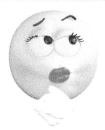

With over thirty years of working with people, I am assuming most readers are tight in
their chest and weaker in their back, this is consistent with the huge numbers of clients I
have seen over the years. I am also assuming a muscle imbalance between the muscles
that affect the scapula; resulting in the scapula being drawn up and forward. Based on
these assumptions, I have included a stretch for your chest, and instructions on how to
strengthen your back to help bring the scapula down and towards your vertebrae, where
they should sit naturally.

If you know your shoulder and neck pain is due to you
having the muscles in your back stronger than the chest
muscles, then this exercise is not recommended for you.
Rockclimbers, for example, may fall into this category.

54

Instructions:

Chest Stretch

To stretch the chest.

Stand near a wall or a corner. Lift one arm up so that your elbow lifts to shoulder height.

Place your elbow on the wall or corner, and bend your elbow to ninety degrees. Turn your body away from your arm.

To increase the intensity of the stretch, turn your head away from the midline of your body.

To change the focus of the stretch, move your arm slightly higher or lower than your shoulder.

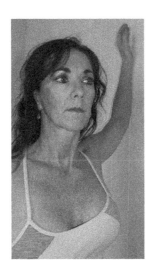 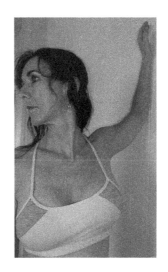

Perform each stretch for at least sixty seconds. Move to the range where you feel a stretch, hold it there gently for one to two seconds, relax off the pressure then repeat.

Once you have stretched what is tight, (your chest), you can then start strengthening what is weak (your upper back).

Generally the mid and lower trapezius, rhomboids, and serratus anterior muscles are the culprits for insufficient strength around the scapula.

If the scapulae don't sit where they are supposed to, generally they come forward. This then affects the spinal curves and creates potential for injury.

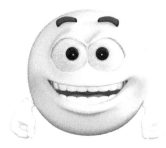

Having the scapula sit correctly, will help create ideal spinal alignment with reduced risk of injury.

Ideally your scapulae sit close to your vertebrae, and flat on your rib cage.

Your serratus anterior are responsible for keeping the scapula on the rib cage. These muscles are underneath the shoulder blade and on the ribs. They are hard to see on an anatomical diagram. If you look at a well toned human, especially male, you may see the 'finger muscles' on the ribs. These are the serratus anterior muscles. We will not be doing any specific exercise to train the serratus anterior muscles in this back health program. If you find your shoulder blades are winging off your rib cage, I suggest you do some exercises that specifically work these muscles.

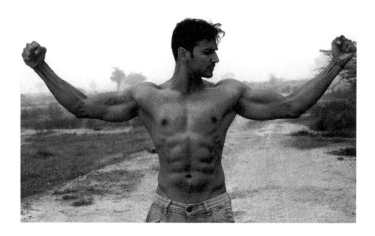

Instructions:

Scapula Control

Lie on the floor on your back. Your legs should be bent, with your spine neutral. Place your arms beside you with your palms up.

This action may seem strange to some readers. This is more than likely because they have not actively contracted these muscles before.

Ensure you are not arching your back or using other muscles. Your neck should stay relaxed and neutral.

Be aware of your shoulder blades touching the floor or mat that you are lying on. Try to activate the muscles in between your scapulae and your vertebrae, your mid and lower trapezius.Use these muscles to try to draw your scapulae down and toward your vertebrae.

Once you are familiar with how to activate these muscles, try to move your arms, while controlling the movement of your scapulae.

Activate your mid and lower trapezius, draw your shoulder blades down and towards your vertebrae. Keep these muscles on. Feel where your scapulae are on the floor or mat, and try to keep them in the same place.

The bottom of your scapulae will move slightly away from your vertebrae.

If you don't consciously contract these muscles your scapulae will move a great deal.

This exercise is intended to teach these muscles to turn on and do their job.

With your scapulae fixed, lift your arms up slowly with your palms facing the ceiling. Once you feel the scapulae move too far or you feel you have lost the control that is desired, return your arms back to the start, with control.

Note: your scapulae will not stay in the same place, they will move. The intention of the exercise, is that you try to restrict the range of movement your scapulae have so you are aware of the muscles that affect your scapulae.

Note: this is not a normal action, but we are trying to teach these muscles to do their job. So when you do use your arms and shoulders, these muscles are able to do their job and help with correct scapula placement and rhythm.

Reset the muscles and repeat the movement. Try to perform ten to fifteen repetitions with correct technique.

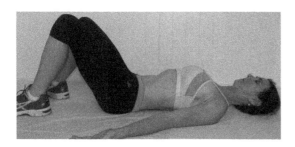 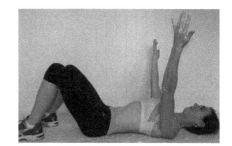

As you become more proficient at controlling the scapulae, you can progress the arm movement to full range.

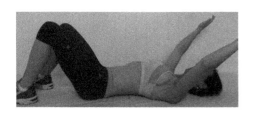 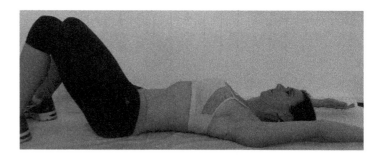

Full range of movement requires you to be able to take your hands up overhead.

As your hands reach the mid point, you need to rotate your arms, so your palms will face the ceiling as you lower.

Only allow your arms to move above your head as far as you can comfortably with your shoulders.

Ensure you do not arch in your back.

Note: I recommend you perform a number of exercises, in this book, with your palms up. The reason behind this is that it allows the muscles in between your shoulder blades to turn on. It encourages ideal posture, and it helps to inhibit the chest muscles from activating and closing the chest; creating poor posture.

This exercise can be done standing. If you do perform it standing, ensure your head is supported, your neck is neutral, and you do not arch your back as you take your arms up. It is a good idea to do it against a wall with your feet slightly away from the wall.

Once you have reached the full range your arms can go to while maintaining neutral spinal alignment, gradually bring your arms back, rotating them at the centre to ensure your palms stay facing up.

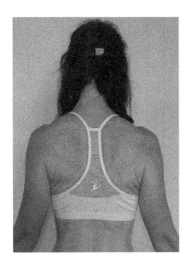 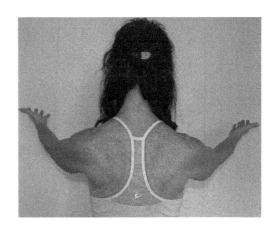

Activate the muscles to draw your shoulder blades down
and together, before you lift your arms up.

Your action should look like this: your shoulders should be open at the chest, your palms should be facing up, your scapulae should draw down and together. Ensure that your spine, including your neck stay relaxed and neutral. Slowly move the arms up, ensuring your palms face the ceiling at all times.

Perform up to fifteen repetitions correctly in one set.

What not to do:

> **Arching the back.**
> **Extending the neck.**
> **Palms down.**

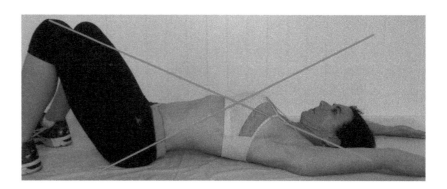

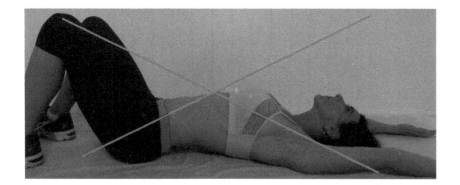

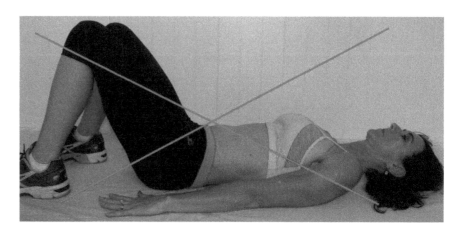

Seated Cobra

This is a progression from 'Scapula Control', but with more load, and it is a more functional movement.

This exercise focuses on activating the muscles across your shoulder blades, including the muscles in the back of your shoulders themselves; including the mid and lower trapezius and the rhomboids..

The action integrates your trunk extensor muscles (muscles that extend your trunk), with the muscles responsible for opening your shoulders, and scapulae retraction (drawing your shoulder blades together). See diagrams 12 and 14.

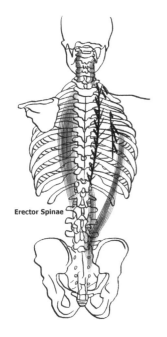

Trunk Extensor Muscles - Erector Spinae

Diagram 13

A lot of people are very 'closed' in their chest and shoulder area. This can then cause a hunching across their shoulders. This may lead to poor shoulder, and poor neck position/posture.

We already know that what happens in one part of the spine directly affects the other parts of the spine. So if you have poor neck posture, it will eventually lead to poor spinal alignment further down the vertebrae.

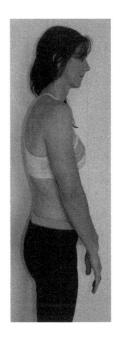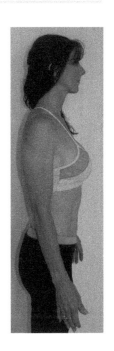

The curves in our spine are supposed to be 'balanced' in that the two lordotic curves will counterbalance the two kyphotic curves. If one is exaggerated one way then the others need to compensate in the opposite direction.

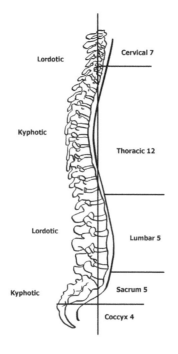

Lordotic

Kyphotic

Lordotic

Kyphotic

Cervical 7

Thoracic 12

Lumbar 5

Sacrum 5

Coccyx 4

Diagram 14

Lordotic and Kyphotic Curves.

Our bodies need these lordotic and kyphotic curves in our spine to help absorb shock going to the brain as we walk and run.

The intention of this exercise is to try to improve the mobility in the thoracic spine, along with the strength and posture in the shoulder girdle area.

It is important to maintain correct spinal alignment at all times throughout this exercise.

If you are aware you fall into a category of postural alignment that is not ideal, try to encourage the ideal curves with all your exercises. You may find that your alignment improves. Your mobility should improve, and this in itself should reduce your pain levels.

Instructions:

Seated Cobra

Sit up straight, on the edge of a chair. Your spine, including your neck, should be neutral.

The space between your chin and your chest should not change throughout the entire movement. Ensure you have activated your deep neck flexors.

Open your shoulders, (externally rotate your shoulders turn your hands out). Your chest should now be open. This position makes it much easier to squeeze your shoulder blades down and together. From here activate your mid and lower trapezius muscles, i.e. the muscles in between and at the bottom of your scapulae.

Activate your core stabilisers.

Slightly exaggerate the drawing down and together of your shoulder blades. Keep these muscles on. While you are doing this, lean forward from your hips.

Your spine should stay neutral and your shoulder blades should not move.

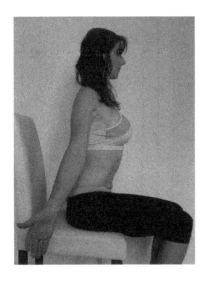

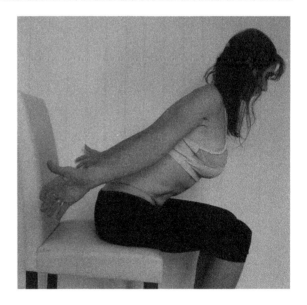

If you notice you are bending in your spine, or losing ideal alignment, you must stop and return to the upright position.

The further forward you lean, causes a greater load on the muscles across your back.

Lean as far forward as you can while keeping your spine neutral.

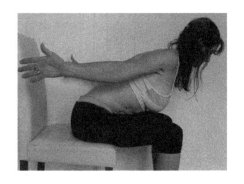

As you become more proficient, mobile, and strong in your back, you should notice your range improves.

When you lean forward try to keep your hands where they started. If you bring your hands forward as you lean forward, you are not working the muscles across your shoulder blades as effectively as you could.

Hold the position for no more than three to five seconds. Return to the start and repeat for at least five to eight correct repetitions, if you can. Remember technique is the determinant of repetitions.

You may start out with shorter holds of one to two seconds. Slowly building up to three to five second holds.

What not to do:

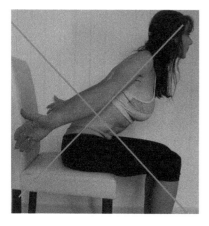
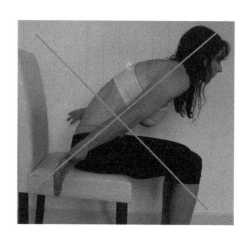

- Extending in the neck
- Rounding in the back
- Flexing too far forward
- Internally rotating the shoulders
- Bringing the hands forward

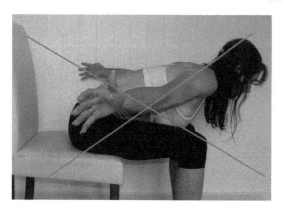
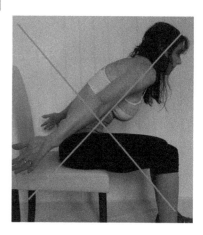

Some readers may need to start this exercise by simply sitting up straight, and opening the chest and shoulders, drawing the scapulae down and together and ensuring that you have correct spinal alignment. As long as you are working in the range that is effective and safe for you, then you should feel improvement in strength, function, and reduced pain levels.

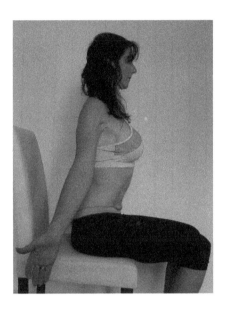 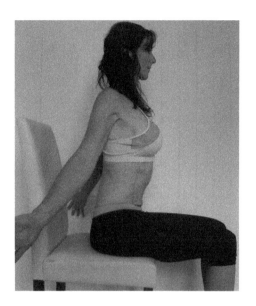

The progression is that you start to lean forward from your hips. You may find that you can only lean one to two degrees to begin with. As long as you are performing the action correctly, it will be of benefit to you. If you allow your back to hunch over, the exercise will not be effective, and you may cause further injury and pain to your back.

You should predominately feel this exercise across your shoulder blades, as well as the muscles down your back.

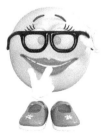

Lots of people tend to hold their breath doing this! Try not to hold your breath.

Prone Hold on Knees (Plank)

Prone Hold on Feet

The purpose of doing this exercise is to teach our TrA what to do. It is also to make us aware of how our TrA function.

The 'Transverse Abdominis Activation' and 'Supine Alternate Leg Lift' exercises have shown you how to activate your TrA muscles. This exercise teaches you how to activate these muscles with a decent load.

The muscles that stabilise your vertebrae, which include TrA and multifidis, stay active for up to ten seconds at a time.

This is imperative to remember.

These core stabiliser muscles need to have at least a one-second rest before they reactivate.

After ten seconds you are still able to hold the plank position, because other muscles, such as your obliques are doing the job. However, if you look closely at your spine, you will notice it is 'sagging' and this indicates a compromise in your spinal stability.

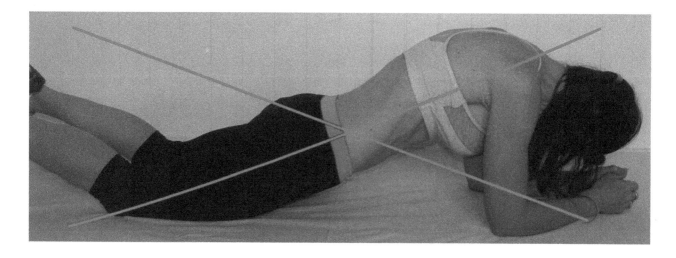

The purpose of this exercise is to improve spinal stability, and core strength, so I recommend you hold this position for no more than ten seconds at a time. Relax and repeat.

You may find initially, that you are able to hold for less than ten seconds before your spinal stability is compromised. If this is the case, stop the exercise. Relax and repeat.

You need to be aware of when your spinal stabilisers cease supporting your vertebrae. Generally, you will feel soreness in your vertebrae. As soon as you notice this, you must stop the exercise.

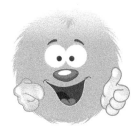

Instructions:

Prone Hold on Knees (Plank)

Prone Hold on Feet

Lie on your stomach. Place your elbows directly below your shoulders. Your neck should be neutral.

> While lying on your stomach, and your elbows on the floor, perform your 'Pelvic Floor Transverse Abdominis Activation' exercise.
>
> You should notice when you activate your pelvic floor and activate your TrA, that your stomach reduces its contact with the floor. (It is very easy to notice if you do this on a cold floor!).

Very gradually progress this exercise by pulling your abdominals in and continue with the 'lifting', You should notice that your pelvis gently lifts off the floor.

Your pelvis should lift off the floor so your knees, hips and shoulders form a straight line.

Note: Your knees should be on the floor.

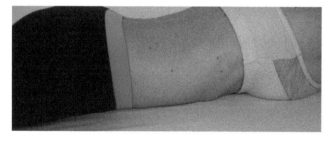 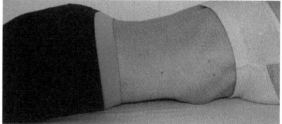

Activate the TrA then lift the pelvis off the floor

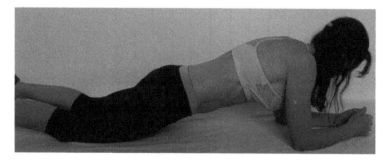

> Hold this position for two to five seconds and be very conscious of how your vertebrae feel.
>
> Slowly lower your pelvis to the floor and then relax your TrA.
>
> Repeat. Activate your core musculature, then lift your pelvis off the floor again. Lower down to the floor then relax the muscles.

If you are doing this correctly, you will not feel anything in your vertebrae. This means you can lift your pelvis higher and progress to the actual exercise.

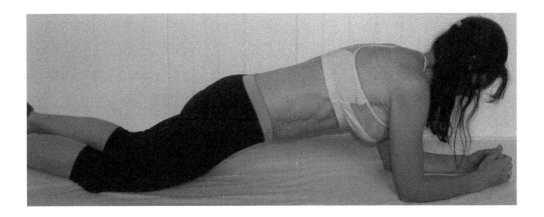

If you do feel it in your vertebrae, it indicates your TrA and multifidis are not activating sufficiently to stabilise your spine. If this is the case, you need to regress to the previous exercises until your muscle contractions are more definite and effective.

Activate your pelvic floor and your TrA. Continue with the drawing in, and lift your pelvis off the floor. Ensure that your spine is neutral. Hold for no more than ten seconds. Lower down, relax, repeat.

If you feel nothing in your vertebrae once you have reached the ten-second hold do not increase the length of the hold. You need to lower down, relax and repeat. This ensures good spinal stability. The number of repetitions is what will cause the overload of the correct muscles, not the duration of the hold.

Be mindful of the length of time these muscles stay activated for; it may vary on different days. At all times you must be very conscious of how your vertebrae feel. If you notice they are feeling sore, then you must lower down, irrespective of the time.

By exercising these muscle groups this way, you are more likely to achieve better back health, and better core strength, than if you tried to hold this position for minutes at a time.

I see so many people perform this exercise incorrectly and I have even heard trainers yelling words of motivation when people are holding this position for as long as they can 'Feel it in your back'. Of course they will feel it in their back. They are actually damaging their spine.

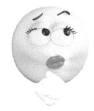

I have heard people commenting they can hold this position for up to thirteen minutes. I can't imagine what this is doing to their spine.

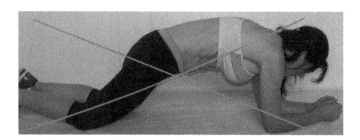

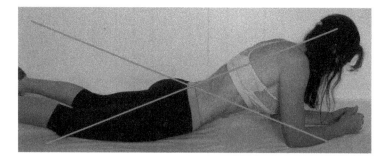

The most important factors for determining your repetitions, your sets, your exercise duration (your hold duration), is the ten second rule and your body. If you feel pain in your vertebrae, you must stop before you reach the ten seconds.

Checklist:

Never hold for more than ten seconds. Never cross your feet.

Ensure correct spinal alignment at all times. Continue to breathe gently and methodically.

The progression is to do the same exercise on your toes, instead of your knees.

There is a marked difference between doing this exercise on your knees and doing it on your feet. You may find you need to reduce the length of the hold initially until the strength in your core musculature builds up.

Your feet should be about hip width apart. Your elbows should be directly below your shoulders. Your spine should remain neutral. Hold for no more than ten seconds at a time.

Note: It is easier to do the plank on your hands and feet, rather than your elbows and your feet.

When doing this exercise it can be made slightly easier by consciously contracting your quads (muscles in the front of the thigh), and your gluteals (your butt muscles). This is because when both of these muscles contract it 'fixes' the pelvis. This then gives the abdominal musculature a solid base to pull from.

If you find you cannot hold the correct position on your feet for the full ten seconds, you can swap between feet and knees for up to ten seconds. For example if you can hold the correct position on your feet for three seconds, simply lower on to your knees for the remaining seven seconds. Alternatively, you can lift back up on to your feet before ten seconds is complete. So you may start on your feet for three seconds, lower on to your knees for four seconds, and then lift up on to your feet again for the last three seconds.

Doing it this way, you are gradually building up muscle endurance in your core musculature, without compromising your spinal stability.

Sets and repetitions are determined by your technique. This means that when you notice you are fatiguing and cannot perform the exercise properly you must cease the exercise. With this exercise, ten seconds should be your limiting factor for every repetition.

Do not aim to hold the same contraction for minutes at a time. It is not ideal for your spinal stability. The variable you can increase is the number of repetitions. Initially, aim for three to six repetitions of ten seconds each. Then gradually build up to eight to ten repetitions of ten seconds, as one set.

Supine Leg Lift Single Leg (Dead Bug)

This is a progression from 'Supine Alternate Leg Lift'. Do not progress to this exercise until you are able to perform that exercise correctly.

The intention of this exercise is to teach your core musculature to stabilise your pelvis, your vertebrae, and your shoulder girdle, while you move your arms and legs.

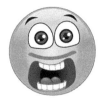

Remember the analogy of the sprinter previously described. You want to move like that. Nothing moves in your trunk, while you move your arms and legs.

This exercise not only works on core strength and stability, it also trains and reinforces a motor engram (movement pattern). Ideally you will teach your body to move both arms and legs while your spine stays fixed and neutral. This movement pattern should transfer to when you are in an upright position, such as walking. When you are upright, your spine is unsupported, so there is a higher risk of injury to your back. This supine position allows you to teach your muscles to stabilise your vertebrae while they are supported, and therefore reduces the risk of injury.

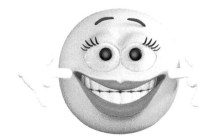

At this stage you should have learned how to activate your deep core stabilisers, your deep neck flexors, the muscles that control your shoulder blades, the muscles that control your pelvis, along with other muscles that all work together to stabilise your trunk and either prevent or assist with movement, depending on the action performed.

This exercise requires integration of some of these muscles, so they work together to create the desired action.

Instructions:

Supine Leg Lift Single Leg (Dead Bug)

Start with lying on your back, and your spine neutral. Your legs should be bent to ninety degrees.

Lift both legs off the floor and ensure your spine stays neutral. Do not allow your spine to flatten on to the floor.

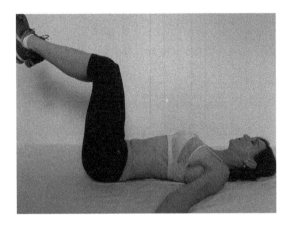

Spine neutral

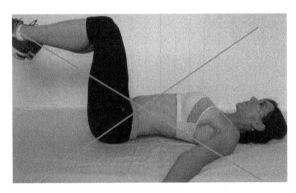

Spine arched

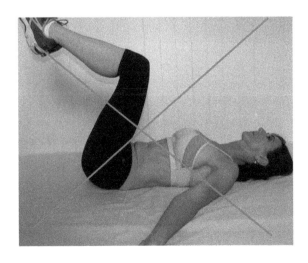

Spine flattened

Ensure your core stabilisers are activated.

Move your left arm and your right leg in opposite directions. The angle at your knee should stay fixed. You are simply moving from your hip joint.

Ensure that your spine stays neutral, i.e. your back does not arch. Your pelvis should not tilt or twist. Your shoulder girdle should not move. Your neck should be totally relaxed and neutral.

Return to the start position, and change to your right arm and your left leg.

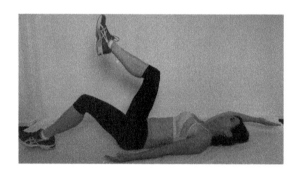 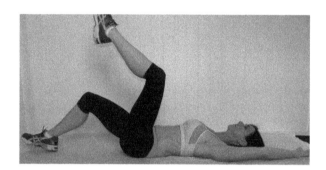

As you get stronger, you can increase the angle at your knee, to increase the load on your core musculature.

The same conditions apply; as soon as you feel your spine come off the floor, or you feel your pelvis tilting, or you have compromised your posture, you must return to the start position.

You should find that as you perform the exercise correctly, your strength improves, your technique improves, and the communication between your brain and your muscles becomes more definite.

Soon enough, your range will improve.

When performing the exercise, as soon as you notice you are doing something incorrect, stop, relax, then try it again. Build up to three minutes in total. This may be made up of ten second repetitions or the length of time that you can perform the action correctly.

If you can perform the exercise correctly continuously for three minutes at a time, then you are able to progress to performing the exercise with straighter legs.

This is a gradual progression and there are many options of angles your knee can stay at. Just straightening your leg by ten to fifteen degrees will have a huge impact on the load you are lifting. Find the angle that challenges you without placing your spine at any risk of injury.

The ultimate progression for this exercise is with your leg straight, but not locked out.

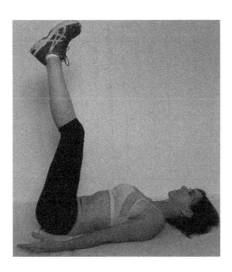

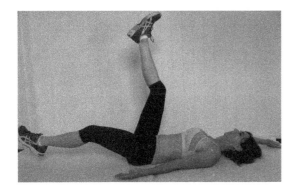
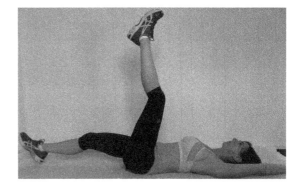

Note: I recommend you move at the hip joint to mimic the walking action. This is why I suggest you keep your knee fixed and do not start with it bent then move it out to straight.

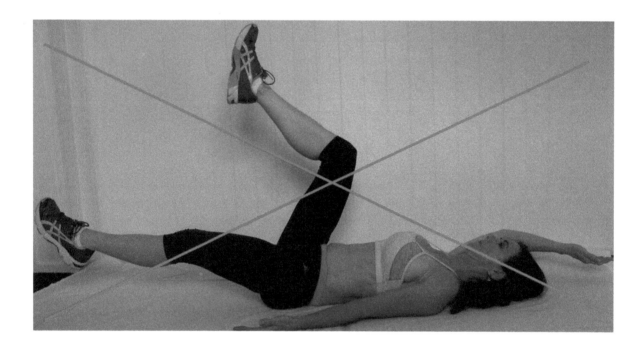

We are training the neuromuscular system at all times and we want to ingrain correct motor patterns so when you move-and-do in daily life, your brain and muscles know exactly what to do properly.

I have found that performing the exercise this way (bent leg to straight leg), a lot of people get injured. The load is increasing too fast for them and they are not able to control their spine as well as when they simply pivot at the hip joint.

Supine Leg Lift Double Leg (Dead Bug)

This is a direct progression from 'Supine Leg Lift Single Leg'. Once you can perform that exercise correctly with straight legs, then you can progress to this.

This exercise is much harder than using just a single leg, so be very aware of your spine position and your trunk posture.

Start with lying on your back, and your spine neutral. Ensure that your legs are bent to ninety degrees.

Lift both legs off the floor and ensure your spine stays neutral; do not allow it to flatten onto the floor.

Lift both arms up so that your hands are pointing to the ceiling. Ensure your core stabilisers are activated.

Move your left arm and both legs at the same time. The angle at your knees should stay fixed; i.e. you are moving at the hip joint only.

Ensure your spine stays neutral, that your back does not arch, that your pelvis does not tilt or twist, that your shoulder girdle does not move, and that your neck is totally relaxed.

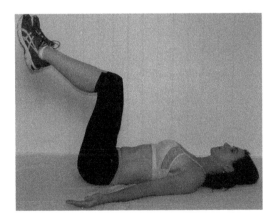 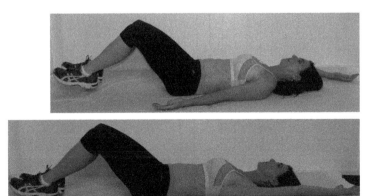

The same conditions apply as for the other exercises; as soon as you feel your spine come off the floor, or you feel your pelvis is tilting, or you have compromised your posture, you must return to the start position.

You should find that as you perform the exercise correctly your strength improves, and your technique should improve due to the communication between your brain and your muscles becoming more definite.

As you become stronger you should be able to increase the angle of your knee, that is your lever length, and therefore the resistance lifted.

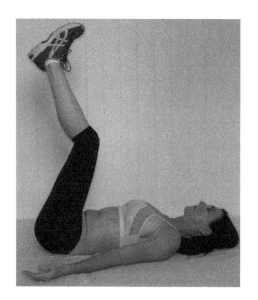
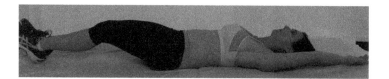
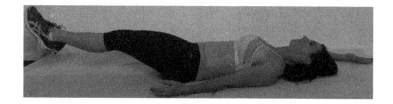

Note: I have seen this exercise done at speed with people's arms anchored overhead and a partner pushing the feet down to the floor. This is fine to do if you have excellent core strength, your spine does not move, and you feel nothing in your back. The majority of the population do not have the necessary core strength to do this properly. When people do this exercise at speed, the potential for causing injury to one's spine increases dramatically.

As you get stronger, you will be able to progress to movements at speed, but this is one exercise I do not recommend most people perform at speed, until you are confident you are able to perform the exercise correctly.

Again, your sets and reps are determined by your technique. Aim for a continuous movement for up to three minutes. This may need to be broken down into smaller time frames, of perhaps fifteen seconds, then rest. Whatever you need to do, in order to do the exercise properly.

Supine Hip Extension Alternate Leg Lift

This is a progression from 'Supine Hip Extension/Prone Hip Extension', do not progress to this exercise until you can execute that exercise correctly.

The progression used in this exercise is the lifting of the leg. Each time a leg is lifted, the base of support (two feet on the floor, to one foot on the floor) changes.

The intention of this exercise is to teach the muscles in and around your pelvic girdle to stabilise your pelvis when you are on one leg.

The action you are performing is not exactly mimicked with walking, but it is very similar in that you have a large load to accommodate. The weight of your pelvis can be very heavy. It is very easy to see if your gluteals are doing their job from this position.

Even though you are in a different position to walking, the idea is to alternate leg lifts as you would do with walking. The chance of creating a new, safer, and more effective motor pattern, is higher, and hopefully, faster.

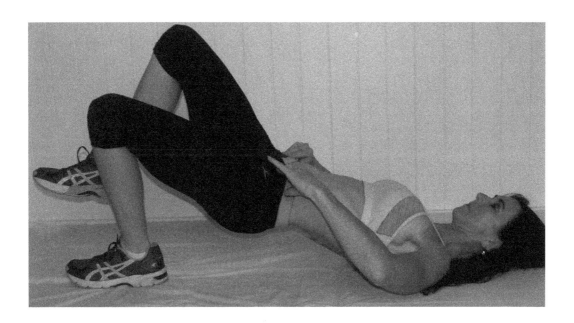

79

Instructions:

Supine Hip Extension Alternate Leg Lift

Lie on your back. Your spine and pelvis should be neutral, with your legs bent, and your feet hip width apart.

Activate your pelvic floor and TrA. Tilt your pelvis backward. (Imagine there is a bowl of water in your pelvis and you are tipping it out on the floor).

This tilting backward of your pelvis places your back muscles on stretch. This then makes it hard for these muscles to turn on.

Keep your core musculature activated. Then consciously activate your gluteals, and try to lift your pelvis off the floor one vertebra at a time.

You may find your hamstrings (muscles at the back of your thigh), cramp. If this is the case, simply lift your toes off the floor.

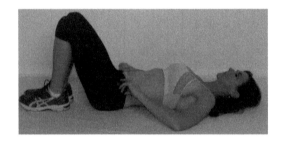

Ensure your gluteals are on. You may feel your lower back muscles are active, but hopefully they are not primarily responsible for the lifting of the hips. Feel both muscle groups (your gluteals and your lower back). The easiest way to tell if a muscle is active, is to feel it. If the muscle feels like it has gone hard, then generally it is active.

Lift up until your knees, hips, and shoulders form a straight line, or just before your back arches (goes into extension), whichever you reach first.

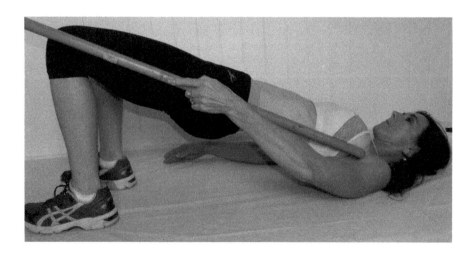

Once you have reached this point, try to lift your left foot off the floor.
Ideally your pelvis and your spine stay neutral throughout the movement.

Place that foot back down and lower your hips to the floor.

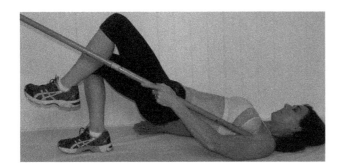
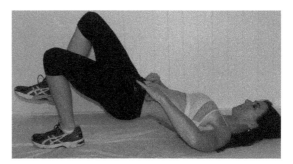

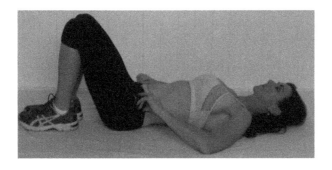

Return to neutral and lift your pelvis off the
floor again. This time, lift your right foot off the
floor. Ideally your pelvis and your spine stay
neutral throughout the movement.

Some readers will notice that lifting one leg is more difficult
than lifting the other; and the pelvis may want to drop or twist.
Try to persist with doing the exercise correctly. This indicates
a muscle imbalance in the gluteals.

You do not need to lift your foot high, it just needs to come off
the floor.

The gluteals of the weight bearing leg must activate to stabilise the pelvis.

You can place your fingers on your pelvis to feel if there is any movement of
the pelvis. Another option is to place a stick across your pelvis to help you
see if there is any movement of the pelvis.

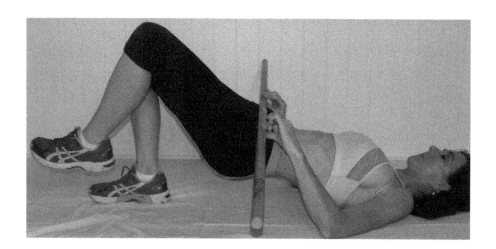

You may find that simply taking most of the weight off one foot is enough to create the tilting in the pelvis. If this is the case, do not lift the foot off the floor. Start with transferring the weight from one foot to the other as if you intend on lifting the foot up, but don't.

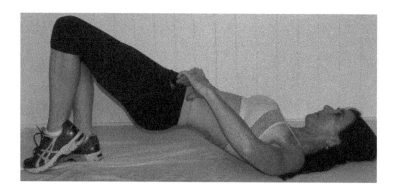

The most important factors to keep in mind here are that the correct muscles are firing to lift your pelvis, and that your pelvis stays horizontal at all times throughout the exercise.

Once you can lift each foot off the floor and keep your pelvis fixed, with the lowering of the pelvis in between, you are then ready to progress.

This time, lift your pelvis, keep it up while you lift one leg, then lower it, then lift the other leg and lower it, then lower your pelvis back to the floor.

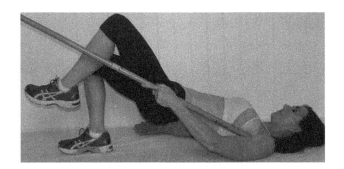 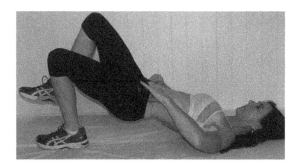

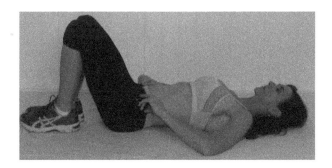

Repeat the exercise for up to ten repetitions, as long as your technique is correct.

Remember: the lifting and lowering of the pelvis one vertebra at a time is essential to the success of this exercise; as is the importance of the pelvis staying horizontal.

Perform eight to twelve repetitions as long as each and every repetition is correct.

Prone Lying Cobra

This is a progression from the 'Seated Cobra'. Once you can perform the 'Seated Cobra' correctly, you can do this exercise.

This is an integration of the muscles that make up our posterior chain, i.e. the muscles that are in the back of our body. These include the trunk extensors, gluteals, hamstrings, and all the muscles across your shoulder girdle. Many more muscles are also being used as you will find out.

The sequence of muscle activation for this exercise is extremely important. You have been instructed on correct activation of the necessary muscle groups, so execution of this exercise should be achievable for you.

If you have not mastered the activation of the muscles from the previous exercises in this book, do not perform this exercise.

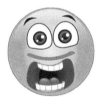

Instructions:

Prone Lying Cobra

Lie prone (face down) on the floor, or a solid surface.

Your feet should be relaxed and they should remain on the floor.

Your spine should stay neutral, with your hands down by your side, and your palms on the floor.

Activate your deep neck flexors. Activate your core stabilisers. Activate your gluteals. Open your chest and draw your shoulder blades down and together. Activate your mid and lower traps. Activate your trunk extensors, then lift and extend your back, so your chest comes off the floor.

Ideally, your neck remains neutral throughout the exercise and your feet remain relaxed on the floor.

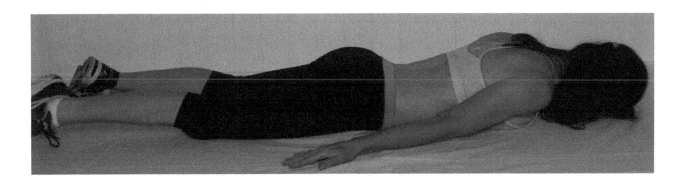

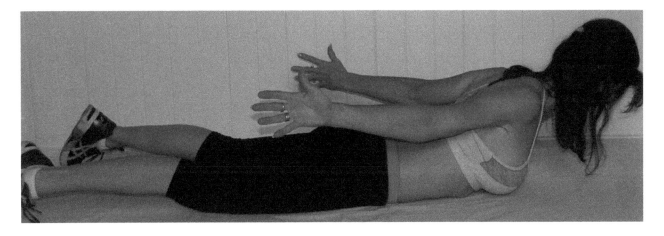

Lift and hold the contraction for no more than two to five seconds.
Lower down, relax and repeat the exercise.

Ensure you continue to breathe while you are doing this exercise.

Note: start with your palms on the floor and when you open your chest, your thumbs will lift straight to the ceiling and your palms will face away from you.

Focus on the opening of the chest, (i.e. external rotation of the shoulders), then the drawing down and together of the scapulae.

The amount of extension you achieve in your lower back is determined purely by the range and strength you have. Do not try to lift higher by compromising your neck alignment.

Perform eight to twelve repetitions as long as each and every repetition is correct.

If you find it difficult to lift your trunk off the floor initially, then simply start with this modified version.

Activate your deep neck flexors. Activate your core stabilisers. Activate your gluteals. Open your chest and draw your shoulder blades down and together. Activate your mid and lower traps. Activate your trunk extensors. Imagine you are lifting your chest off the floor, but don't actually do it.

Relax and repeat.

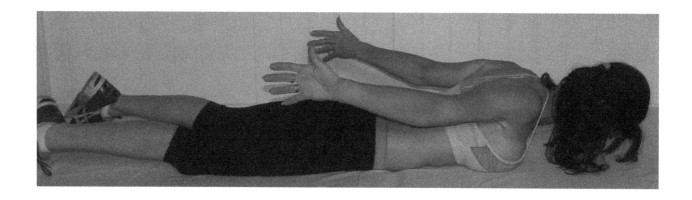

Your neck must stay in neutral. Your feet must stay on the floor.

Activating your gluteals is essential, because it helps to stabilise the pelvis and allows the lower back muscles to have a solid base to pull from.

Ensure you are turning your hands the correct way. Do not internally rotate your shoulders.

What not to do:

Extending the neck

Palms up on the floor

Internal rotation of the shoulders

Lifting the feet of the floor

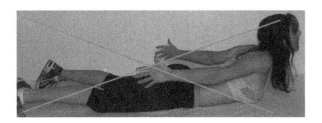
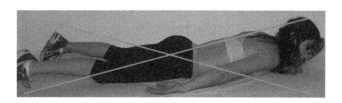

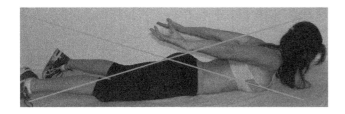
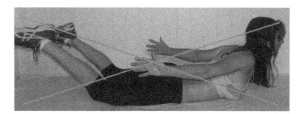

The Clam

This exercise is often executed using the wrong muscles. It is important to be aware of what you are doing and why. That is the purpose of this book to teach you what you need to work, why, and how.

Just as we have been working the deep stabilisers of the neck and trunk, we also need to work the deep stabilisers, and external rotators of the hip.

These muscles include: the piriformis, superior gemellus, inferior gemellus, obturator internus, obturator externus and quadratus femoris, otherwise known as the 'Deep Six'.

When you see where these muscles are located it should be easy to see where you should feel the muscle activation with the clam exercise.

Try to ensure this is where you do feel it.

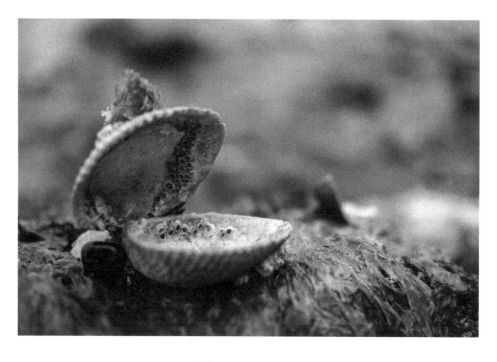

External Rotators of the Hip - 'The Deep Six Muscles'

Diagram 15 a & b

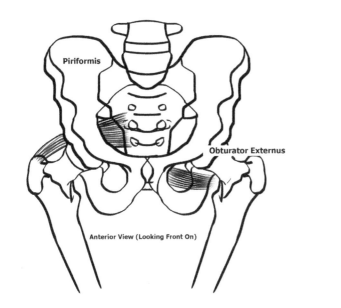

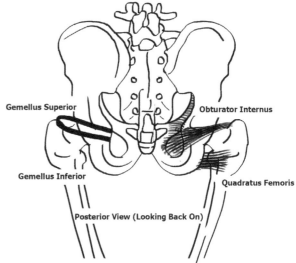

Instructions:

The Clam

Lie on your side with your legs on top of each other. Ensure your hips are bent to approximately seventy degrees at the hip. Your feet should be in line with your trunk. Your spine should be neutral; including your neck.

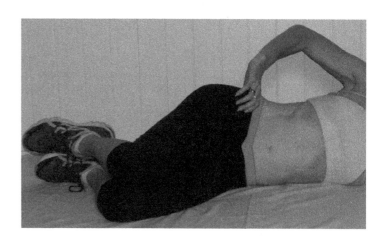

If you move your knees further away from your body, i.e. increase the angle of the hip joints, then you tend to work the lower portion of the deep six muscles more so. Generally it is thought that the upper portion of the deep six muscles are weaker, so it is recommended to bend the knees to seventy degrees or less, i.e. bring the knees closer up to the body.

Support your head so your neck is neutral. Ensure your spine stays neutral.

Palpate (feel) the sitting bone of the top hip. Feel just under this bone, and as you open your top leg up you should feel the muscles under your fingers go hard. This should be your quadratus femoris activating.

This exercise is not designed to activate your gluteus maximus. If performed correctly, you should be activating your deep six stabiliser muscles of your hip, as named above.

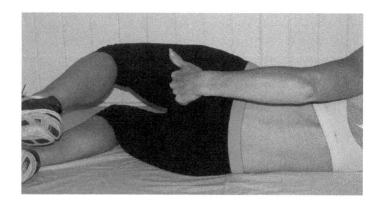

You should only be able to lift your top leg no more than forty five degrees. If you lift it further you are not activating the correct muscles, and/or you are allowing the pelvis to rock back. This is not ideal.

Ensure your pelvis does not move as you lift the top leg.

Perform up to twenty repetitions correctly. Relax and change legs.

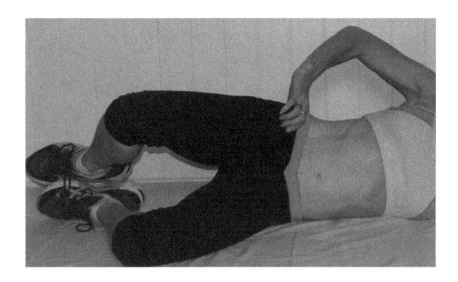

If you notice one leg is noticeably weaker than the other, work that one first, then the stronger leg, then the weaker leg again.

The intention is to have equal strength, range, and function with both hips.

Once you have mastered the correct muscle activation and you have equal strength on both sides, you can progress. Your progression is simply putting a weight on your bent knee.

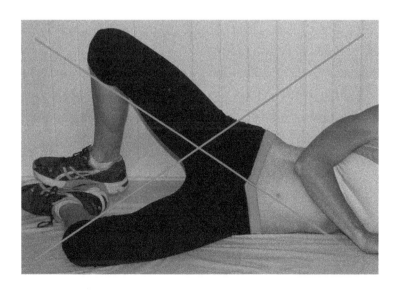

Trendelenberg Standing

This is named after the test that can be performed to see if someone is strong enough in the muscles of their pelvis that keep it horizontal when standing on one leg.

To perform the test, simply lift one foot off the floor. If you notice your pelvis drop on the opposite side, then you have a positive Trendelenburg.

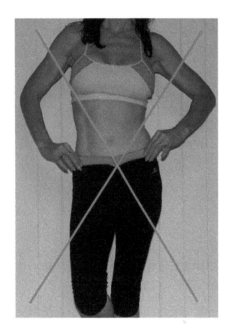 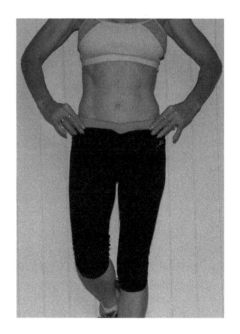

Basically this means that the muscles that support the pelvis are not strong enough to stabilise the pelvis when standing on one leg. If you think about the walking action, we spend approximately sixty percent of walking on one leg.

The complications of this can be enormous. When we stand on one leg in the walking (gait) phase, it is possible to experience up to three times more load on the hip joint, compared to when standing on two legs.

If you look at the pelvis and its connection to the vertebrae, it should be apparent that when the pelvis tilts, it affects the vertebrae. Every step taken with a positive Trendelenburg causes tilting and pivoting in the vertebrae.

Over time, this can cause pain, dysfunction and injury.

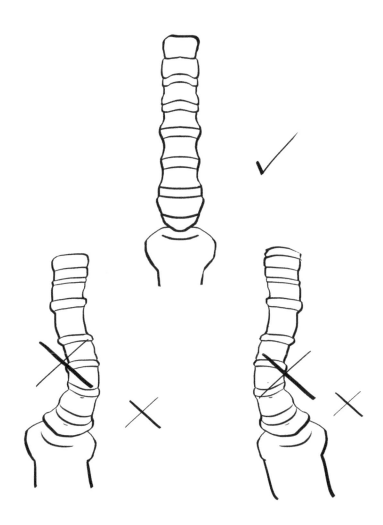

Instructions:

Static Trendelenburg

Stand in front of a mirror so you can see your pelvis. Ensure your spine is neutral, and your pelvis is horizontal.

Place your fingers (or some markers) on the same point on each side of your pelvis, preferably a bony point.

Activate your core stabilisers. Lift one foot off the floor. Ensure your pelvis stays horizontal.

Hold that leg off the floor for up to ten to thirty seconds. Change legs. Repeat this activity on each leg three to four times.

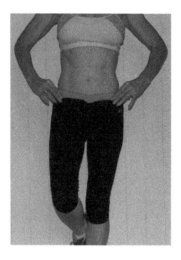

You may find that when you hold your leg up, you notice you start to fatigue in the muscles that stabilise the pelvis. If you see your pelvis dropping, try to keep it horizontal for the set amount of time. Focus on 'carrying the load' in the hip abductors (gluteus medius and minimus).

Diagram 17
Contributors to Pelvic Stability

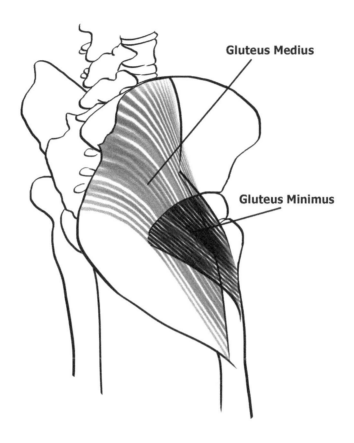

Gluteus Medius

Gluteus Minimus

Compare limbs. If there is a significant difference between
left and right, you need to work to make both legs the
same. At the same time, you need to work to ensure the
pelvis does not move or drop when you lift either leg.

**Once you are able to prevent the dropping of your
pelvis with your leg lifted, you can progress to
'Dynamic Trendelenburg'.**

Instructions:

Dynamic Trendelenburg Alternate Leg Lift

Stand in front of a mirror so you can see your pelvis. Ensure your spine is neutral, and your pelvis is horizontal.

Place your fingers (or some markers) on the same bony point on each side of your pelvis.

Activate your core stabilisers. Lift one foot off the floor. Ensure your pelvis stays horizontal. Hold the foot off the floor for no more than two complete seconds, then lower that leg, and lift the other leg. This very closely mimics walking, however, the leg is lifting higher than in a normal gait pattern.

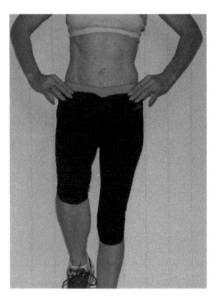 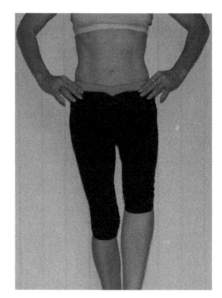

This is very similar in action to the static exercise, but the movement is much more fluid.

You should be constantly moving, but with control. Lift and lower one leg, then lift and lower the other, continuously. The pelvis must stay horizontal.

You may find the transition with changing legs is the most difficult stage to keep the pelvis horizontal. Focus on the pelvis and try to keep it fixed.

Focus on 'carrying the load' in the hip abductors (gluteus medius and minimus).

Try to lift and lower alternate legs for a total of three minutes. Remember technique is your determinant of repetitions, sets, and time.

Instructions:

Dynamic Trendelenburg Lift and Lower Pelvis

Stand in front of a mirror so you can see your pelvis. Ensure your spine is neutral, and your pelvis is horizontal.

Place your fingers (or some markers) on the same bony point on each side of your pelvis.

Activate your core stabilisers. Lift one foot off the floor. Allow your pelvis to drop on the other side then using your hip abductors (gluteus medius and minimus) lift your pelvis up past horizontal.

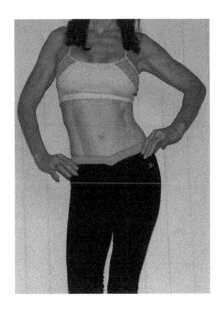 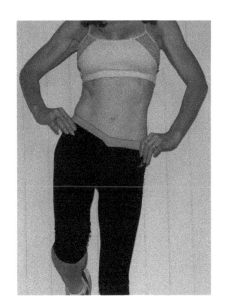

Try to keep your spine neutral. Ensure it is your pelvis lifting and lowering, not just your knee bending.

You should feel the muscles turning on in the side of your pelvis.

Try to lift and lower for up to thirty seconds. Relax and repeat. Perform the exercise for a total of three minutes, if you can, properly.

What not to do:

Bending the weight-bearing knee.
Twisting in the pelvis.

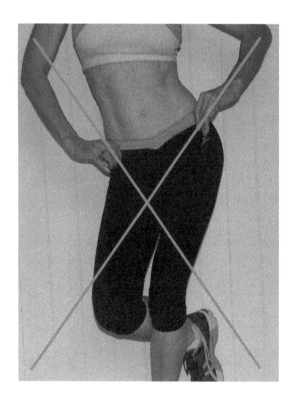 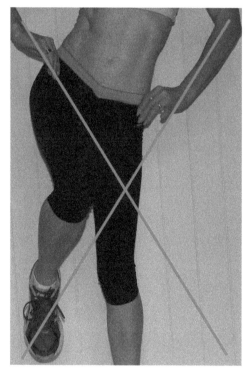

Trendelenberg Lunge Static

This is a progression from the 'Trendelenburg Standing' exercise. This time you are in a lunge position and this places more load on your abductor muscles. If you cannot perform the 'Trendelenburg Standing', do not progress to this exercise.

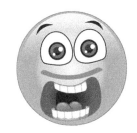

Note: if your knees prevent you from doing a lunge, do not attempt these exercises. Simply stay with the 'Trendelenburg Standing' exercise to strengthen your hip abductor muscles.

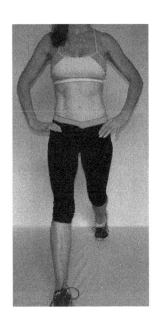

Adopt a lunge position. Imagine you have a plumb line that must pass through the centre of your hip, the centre of your knee, and the second toe of that leg. (This is what is meant by 'hips, knees, and feet in alignment').

This plumb line rule applies to both legs.

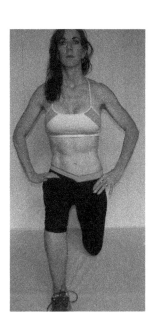

Ensure your pelvis is horizontal. Slowly lower into a lunge position. Ideally your spine remains neutral, and your pelvis remains horizontal.

Hold the lunge position for ten to fifteen seconds if you can. Lift up and repeat using the same leg. If you need a rest from that leg, simply change legs. Ensure you perform the same number of repetitions each leg.

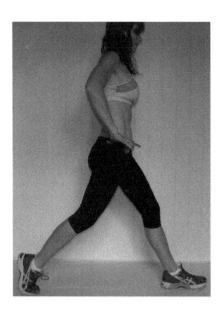
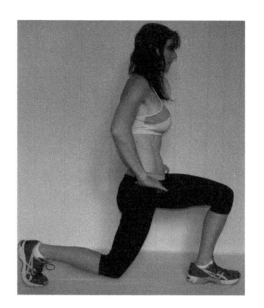

At all times you need to concentrate on your alignment.

Once you are confident you have good pelvic stability with the static lunge, you can progress to the dynamic lunge.

Perform up to eight to ten repetitions per leg, as long as they are performed correctly.

What not to do:

Not keeping the pelvis horizontal.

Not maintaining the plumb line with knees, hips, and feet.

Lunging forward instead of down.

Allowing the knee to move forward of the foot.

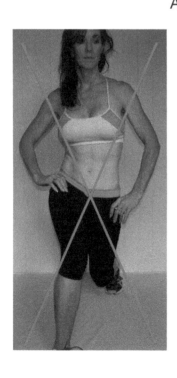
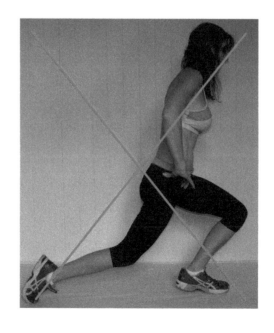

Trendelenberg Lunge Dynamic

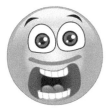

This is a progression from the 'Trendelenburg Standing' exercise. This time you are in a lunge position and this places more load on your abductor muscles. If you cannot perform the 'Trendelenburg Standing', or the 'Trendelenburg Lunge Static', do not progress to this exercise.

Note: if your knees prevent you from doing a lunge, do not attempt this exercise. Simply stay with the 'Trendelenburg Standing' exercise to strengthen your hip abductor muscles.

Adopt a lunge position. Imagine you have a plumb line that must pass through the centre of your hip, the centre of your knee, and the second toe of that leg. (This is what is meant by 'hips, knees, and feet in alignment').

This plumb line rule applies to both legs.

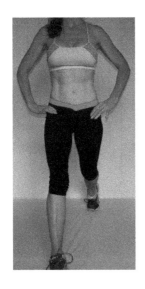
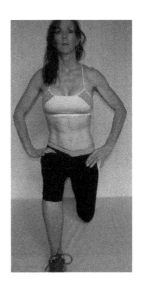

Ensure your pelvis is horizontal and slowly lower into a lunge position. Ideally your spine remains neutral, and your pelvis remains horizontal.

Hold the lunge position for no more than two complete seconds, then slowly lift up to the start position. Lunge down again and repeat for up to fifteen repetitions depending on your technique.

Change legs.

At all times you must concentrate on your alignment.

Note: to perform a lunge your action is that of you lowering your pelvis straight down. The back knee will also move straight down to the floor, and should just miss touching the floor. Your front knee does not move forward of your toes.

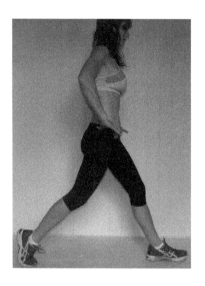 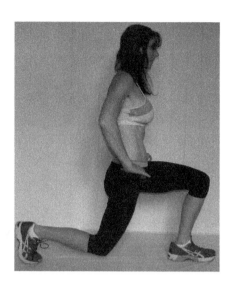

What not to do:

Not keeping the pelvis horizontal.

Not maintaining the plumb line with knees, hips, and feet.

Lunging forward instead of down.

Allowing the knee to move forward of the foot.

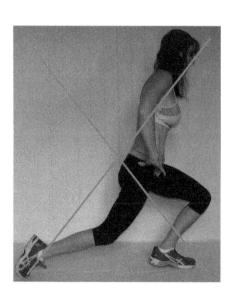 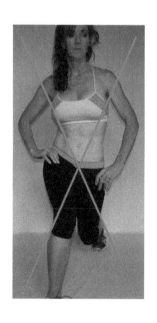

Four-Point Isometric Contraction & Transverse Abdominis Activation

It is ideal when performing these four- point exercises that you have a piece of dowel that you can use.

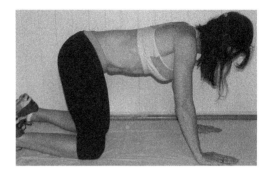

This exercise series is a progression from the other exercises in that your spine is no longer supported. If you have not mastered the other exercises previous to these, I recommend you continue with them, before attempting the four-point series.

Place your hands directly below your shoulders. Place your knees directly below your hips. Note: that your knees are not together, and that your arms are straight but not locked.

If your arms are longer in relation to your thighs, you may need to bend your arms slightly to bring your trunk to a more horizontal position. If your shoulders are much higher than your hips, when you place the dowel along your spine, you may find that the dowel slides off.

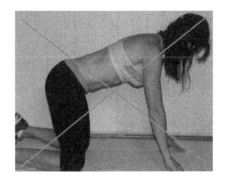

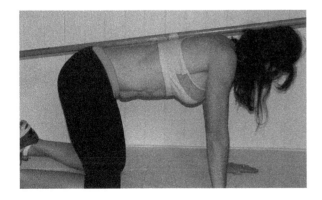

Keep your spine neutral. Place the dowel along your spine. You should have three points of contact; your head, your thoracic spine, and your sacrum.

The dowel should stay fixed along your spine with those three points of contact throughout each exercise.

Your core stabilisers must activate to prevent unwanted movement; tilting, twisting, and lifting of the shoulders and/or hips.

You may notice the dowel rolls off to the same side each time. If this is the case, there is a definite muscle imbalance that needs to be addressed.

Instructions:

Four-Point Isometric Contraction & Transverse Abdominis Activation

> Adopt the four-point position as described above. Place the dowel along your spine.
>
> Ensure you have three points of contact; your head, your thoracic spine, and your sacrum.

Breathe in: You should see your stomach expand.

Breathe out: You should see your stomach come back to its normal resting position. Activate your pelvic floor. You should see no movement.

Activate your TrA. You should see your stomach reduce in size/move toward your spine.

Hold for two to five seconds. Repeat this activity for three minutes.

Ensure you do not move your body at all. It is simply activation of your deep core stabilisers.

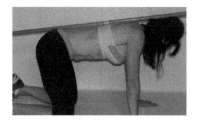 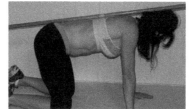 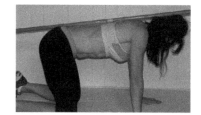

What not to do:

Moving in the trunk when activating the TrA. Not maintaining neutral alignment.

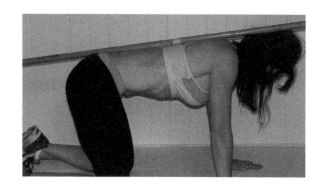

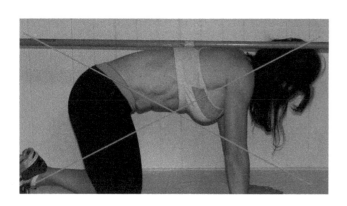

> Once you are confident with this exercise, you can progress to 'Four-Point Progression One: Alternate Arm Lift'.

Four-Point Progression One: Alternate Arm Lift

This is the first progression in the four-point series. Attempt this exercise when you are competent in performing the 'Four-Point Isometric Contraction and Transverse Abdominis Activation'.

Keep your trunk fixed, the dowel along your spine, and lift one hand off the floor.

You must have your core stabilisers on in order to prevent the dowel from rolling off your back.

Adopt the four-point position as described above. Place the dowel along your spine.

Ensure you have three points of contact; your head, your thoracic spine, and your sacrum.

Maintaining the points of contact and therefore the curves in your spine, activate your core stabilisers and your deep neck flexors.

You may notice your body wanting to 'move' or 'adjust' to help perform the action, and this 'moving' or 'adjusting' is not desirable. We need to teach our stabilisers to activate to prevent the movement.

You don't need to lift your arm high, you can just simply lift your hand off the floor. This is changing your base of support and forces your stabilisers to activate to prevent unwanted movement.

Be aware of your three points of contact at all times. They should not change.

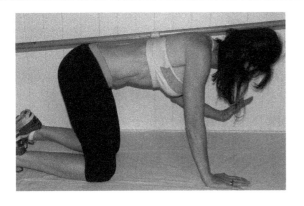 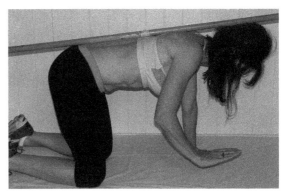

Place that hand back on the floor directly below your shoulder. Then lift the other hand off the floor.

Continue lifting and lowering alternate hands off the floor. At all times think about your spinal curves, the points of contact with the dowel, your deep neck flexors, and your core stabilisers.

Repeat for a number of repetitions; up to three minutes in total. Remember technique is your determining factor in sets, repetitions, and time.

Once you feel confident with simply lifting your hand off the floor, challenge yourself a little more. Make the lever longer, i.e. do the same thing but with your arm straight. A longer lever means a heavier load.

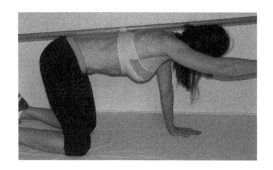 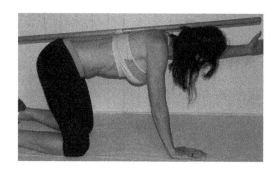

Ensure when you lift your arm, that your thumb points to the ceiling. This is a much safer and more comfortable position for your shoulder joint.

Once you are confident with this exercise, you can progress to 'Four-Point Progression Two: Alternate Leg Lift'.

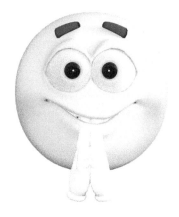

Four-Point Progression 2: Alternate Leg Lift

This is the second progression in the four-point series. Attempt this exercise when you are competent in performing the Four-Point Progression One: Alternate Arm Lift.

Adopt the four-point position as described above. Place the dowel along your spine.

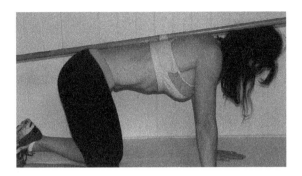

Ensure you have three points of contact; your head, your thoracic spine, and your sacrum.

Maintaining the points of contact and therefore the curves in your spine, activate your core stabilisers and your deep neck flexors.

Keep your trunk fixed, keep the dowel along your spine, and lift one leg off the floor.

You must have your core stabilisers on and your hip stabilisers on, in order to prevent the dowel from rolling off your back.

You may notice the dowel more readily rolls off your body doing this exercise, compared to lifting alternate arms. This is more likely due to the desire for your body to bring your weight over your base of support. Your body will try to bring the unsupported hip over the knee that is on the floor.

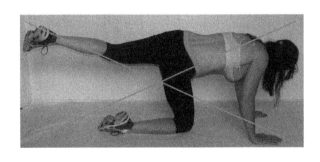

You need to concentrate on activating the hip abductors of the weight bearing leg, so they 'carry the load' properly.

Your technique is important with this exercise. You need to slide your leg backward, not lift it up. To do this, you need to activate your gluteals of the moving leg.

You will need to slide the leg back to its original position, i.e. directly under your hip.

Be aware of your three points of contact at all times with the dowel. They should not change.

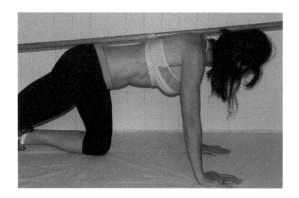 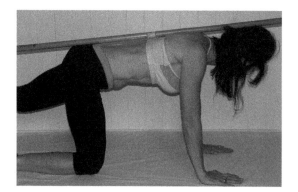

Continue lifting and lowering alternate legs off the floor. At all times think about your spinal curves, the points of contact with the dowel, your deep neck flexors, and your core stabilisers.

Repeat for a number of repetitions; up to three minutes in total. Remember technique is your determining factor in sets, repetitions, and time.

Once you are confident with this exercise, you can progress to 'Four-Point Progression Three: Alternate Arm and Leg Lift'.

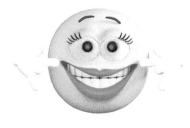

Four-Point Progression Three: Alternate Arm & Leg Lift

This is the third, progression in the four-point series. Attempt this exercise when you are competent in performing the 'Four-Point Progression Two: Alternate Leg Lift'.

Adopt the four-point position as described above. Place the dowel along your spine.

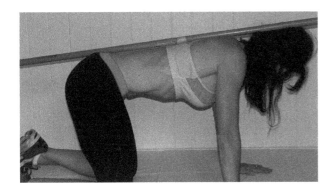

Ensure you have three points of contact; your head, your thoracic spine, and your sacrum.

Maintaining the points of contact and therefore the curves in your spine, activate your core stabilisers and your deep neck flexors.

Keep your trunk fixed, the dowel along your spine, lift your right leg and your left arm off the floor.

In order to prevent the dowel from rolling off your back, ensure your core stabilisers and your hip stabilisers are both on.

Focus on trying to keep the dowel on your spine with your three points of contact. Your spinal curves should remain the same throughout the movement.

All the cues you used for the previous exercises in this series, need to be used to execute the exercise correctly.

Be aware if your body is trying to 'cheat'. What is it doing? What is it wanting to do? What should it be doing? Focus on teaching your body what it is supposed to be doing. It will learn.

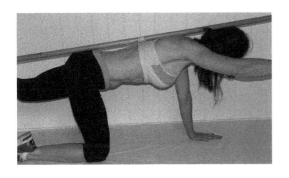

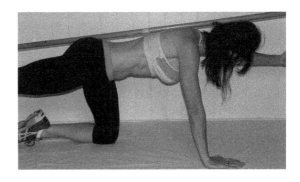

Continue alternating with lifting your opposite arm and leg off the floor.

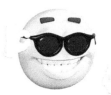

The dowel generally does not allow you to 'cheat'. If you are doing something wrong, the dowel should roll off. This is why I recommend you use it.

Repeat for a number of repetitions; up to three minutes in total. Remember technique is your determining factor in sets, repetitions, and time.

Once you are confident with this exercise, you can progress to 'Four-Point Progression Four: Alternate Arm and Leg Alphabet'.

Four-Point Progression Four: Alternate Arm & Leg Alphabet

This is the fourth, progression in the four-point series. Attempt this exercise when you are competent in performing the 'Four-Point Progression Three: Alternate Arm and Leg Lift'.

Adopt the four-point position as described above. Place the dowel along your spine.

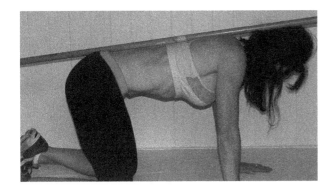

Ensure you have three points of contact; your head, your thoracic spine, and your sacrum.

Maintaining the points of contact and therefore the curves in your spine, activate your core stabilisers and your deep neck flexors.

Keep your trunk fixed, the dowel along your spine, and lift your right leg and your left arm off the floor.

Ensure your core stabilisers and your hip stabilisers are on, in order to prevent the dowel from rolling off your back.

Focus on trying to keep the dowel on your spine with your three points of contact. Your spinal curves should remain the same throughout the movement.

Hold the right leg and left arm off the floor and without moving your trunk, start to write the alphabet with your limbs. Your hand and foot should move in a pattern that forms the shape of the letters.

Keep those two limbs up for no more than thirty seconds, then change to the other arm and leg. Now you should have your left leg and your right arm up.

Gradually progress through the alphabet with both limbs.

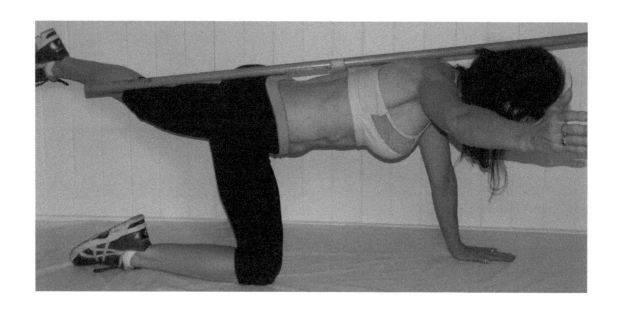

Repeat up to three minutes in total for both
sides. Remember technique is your determining
factor in sets, repetitions, and time.

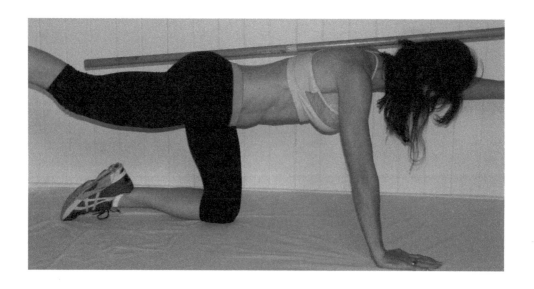

Kneeling Cobra

This is a progression from the 'Prone Lying Cobra'. The exercise is more integrative and functional than lying down on the floor.

This exercise integrates the muscles in our posterior chain, i.e. the muscles that are in the back of our body. These include the trunk extensors, gluteals, hamstrings, and all the muscles across your shoulder girdle. Many more muscles are also being used as you will find out.

The sequence of muscle activation for this exercise is extremely important. You have been instructed on correct activation of the necessary muscle groups, so execution of this exercise should be achievable for you.

If you have not mastered the activation of the muscles from the previous exercises in this book, do not perform this exercise

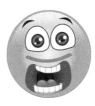

If you cannot kneel for whatever, reason, this exercise can be performed in a standing position.

Instructions:

Kneeling

If you notice you are bending in your spine, you must stop and return to the upright position.

Kneel in an upright position, on the floor. Ensure your spine including your neck are neutral. The space between your chin and your chest should not change throughout the entire movement. Ensure your deep neck flexors and core stabilisers are activated.

Open your shoulders, turn your hands out - i.e. externally rotate your shoulders. Your chest should now be open. This position makes it much easier to squeeze your shoulder blades down and together and activate your mid and lower trapezius muscles.

Activate the muscles (mid and lower trapezius muscles), to draw your shoulder blades down and together, and keep them on.

Hold this muscle activation and lean forward from your hips.

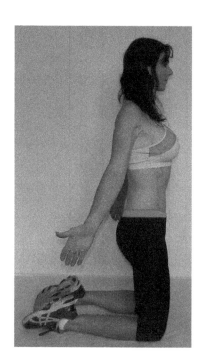

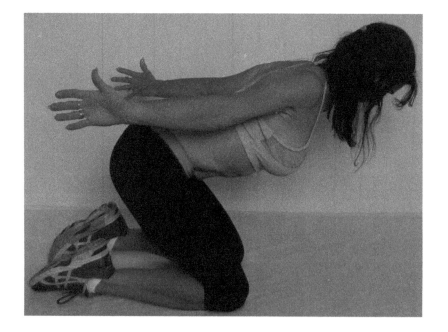

The further forward you lean, the higher the load is on the muscles across your back.

Only lean as far forward as you can while keeping your spine neutral. As you become more proficient, mobile, and strong in your back, you should notice your range improves.

Keep within the range you that you can execute the technique correctly.

As you lean forward try to keep your hands where they started. If you bring your hands forward as you lean forward, you are not working the muscles as effectively as you could.

Hold the position for no more than three to five seconds. Return to the start and repeat for at least five to eight correct repetitions if you can. Remember technique is the determinant of repetitions.

You may start out with shorter holds of one to two seconds. Slowly building up to three to five second holds.

You may find that you can only lean forward one to two degrees to begin with. As long as you are doing it correctly, it will be of benefit to you. If you allow your back to hunch over, the exercise will not be effective, and you may cause further injury and pain to your back.

Build up to eight to twelve repetitions as long as each and every repetition is correct.

Activating your gluteals is essential, because it helps to stabilise the pelvis and allow the lower back muscles a solid base to pull from. Your gluteals should help in returning your trunk to the upright position. Actively squeeze them to help them turn on when you lift your trunk; this will help take the load off your back.

What not to do:

Allowing the back to round forward

Internally rotating the shoulders.

Leading with the chin.

Not activating the gluteals.

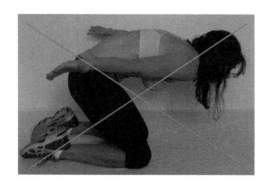
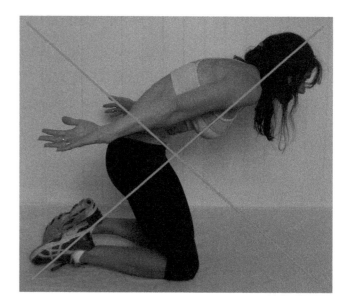

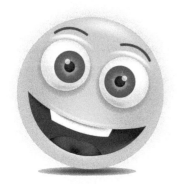

Instructions:

Standing Cobra

Stand up straight. Ensure your spine including your neck is neutral. The space between your chin and your chest does not change throughout the entire movement. Ensure your deep neck flexors and core stabilisers are activated.

Open your shoulders, turn your hands out - i.e. externally rotate your shoulders. Your chest should now be open. This position makes it much easier to squeeze your shoulder blades down and together and activate your mid and lower trapezius muscles.

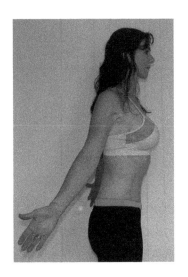

Bend your knees slightly and they should stay fixed at that angle.

Activate the muscles (mid and lower trapezius muscles), to draw your shoulder blades down and together, and keep them on. While you are doing this, lean forward from your hips.

If you notice you are bending in your spine, you must stop and return to the upright position.

The further forward you lean, the higher the load is on the muscles across your back.

Only lean as far forward as you can while keeping your spine neutral. As you become more proficient, mobile, and strong in your back, you should notice your range improves.

Keep within the range you that you can execute the technique correctly.

As you lean forward try to keep your hands where they started. If you bring your hands forward as you lean forward, you are not working the muscles as effectively as you could.

Hold the position for no more than three to five seconds. Return to the start and repeat for at least five to eight correct repetitions if you can. Remember technique is the determinant of repetitions.

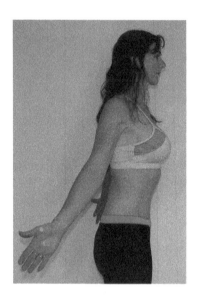 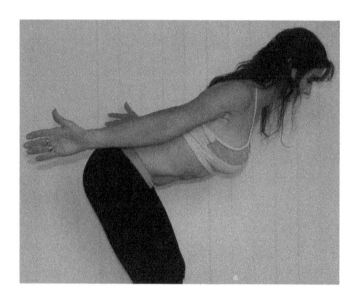

You may start out with shorter holds of one to two seconds. Slowly building up to three to five second holds.

You may find that you can only lean one to two degrees to begin with. As long as you are doing it correctly, it will be of benefit to you. If you allow your back to hunch over, the exercise will not be effective, and you may cause further injury and pain to your back.

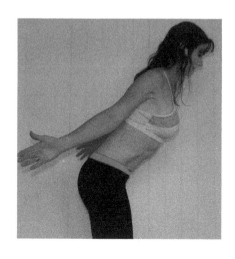

Build up to eight to twelve repetitions as long as
each and every repetition is correct.

**Activating your gluteals is essential, because it helps
to stabilise the pelvis and allow the lower back muscles
a solid base to pull from. Your gluteals should help in
returning your trunk to the upright position. Actively
squeeze them to help them turn on when you lift your
trunk; this will help take the load off your back.**

What not to do:

Allowing the back to round forward.

Internally rotating the shoulders.

Leading with the chin.

Not activating the gluteals.

Four-Point Prone Hold Lift Alternate Leg

This is a direct progression from 'Prone Hold on Knees' and 'Prone Hold on Feet'.

It is also an integration of the Prone Hold exercises as well as the Four-Point Series.

Ensure you do not feel any soreness in your vertebrae at all.

The transfer of weight with each leg lift is what makes the exercise more challenging. You must maintain correct spinal alignment at all times.

Remember to maximise spinal stability and function, hold for no more than ten seconds at a time. Simply lower your knees to the floor, rest for one second then lift again.

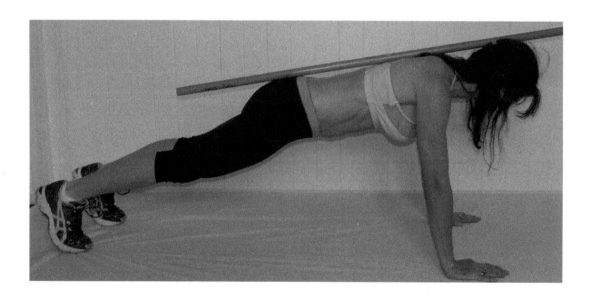

Instructions:

Four-Point Prone Hold Lift Alternate Leg

Adopt a four-point position as shown.

Ensure your spine, including your neck, is neutral. Your feet should be hip width apart, and your hands should be directly below your shoulders.

Ensure your core stabilisers are activated to support your vertebrae. Place the dowel along your spine.

Keep your trunk fixed and lift one foot off the floor. Ensure you use your gluteal muscles to lift that leg.

Lower that leg down and lift the other leg.

Continue to lift alternate legs. Be mindful of the ten second rule. Relax and repeat at each ten second mark or beforehand if you feel anything in your spine.

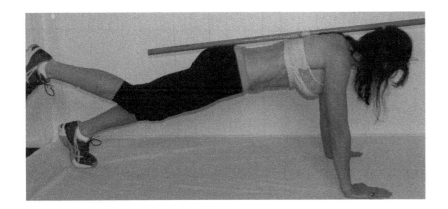

Correct technique is of the utmost importance at all times.

You want to ensure that your ankles, knees, hips, and shoulders form a straight line that does not deviate at all when you move your limbs.

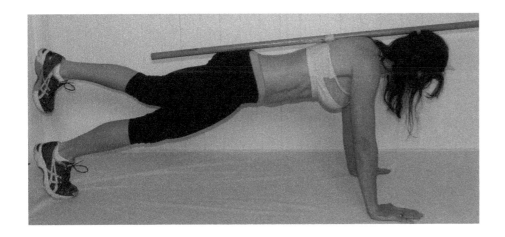

Repetitions, sets, and exercise duration (hold duration), are all determined by your body. If you feel pain in your vertebrae, you must stop. If you are not doing the exercise correctly, you must stop and regress the exercise.

What not to do:

Lifting the pelvis up

Rotating in the trunk or pelvis

Not maintaining spinal stability

Not using your gluteals to extend your leg

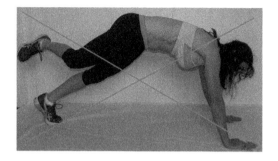

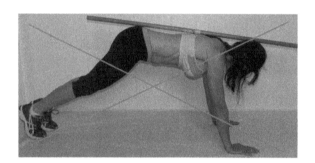

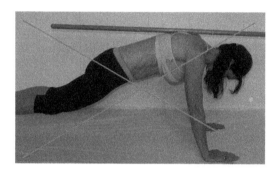

A lot of people will compensate by lifting their pelvis up. This reduces the load on the core stabilisers. It is not ideal.

If you cannot do the exercise without moving your trunk in a compensatory manner, then regress to the previous exercises, until you are stronger.

The next progression is to do the same exercise on your elbows, instead of your hands.

Remember to contract your quads and gluteals to help fix the pelvis.

Do not aim to hold the same contraction for minutes at a time. It is not ideal for your spinal stability. Aim to hold each contraction for ten seconds. The factor you can increase is the number of repetitions. Aim for three repetitions initially. Then gradually build up to eight to ten repetitions.

Four-Point Prone Hold Lift Alternate Hand

This is a direct progression from 'Four-Point Prone Hold Lift Alternate Leg'. Once you can perform that exercise correctly and with confidence, then you can progress to this exercise.

There is a marked difference between doing this exercise; lifting alternate hands, and the previous exercise; lifting alternate feet.

The transfer of weight with the lift of each hand is what makes the exercise more challenging. You must maintain correct spinal alignment at all times.

Remember to maximise spinal stability and function, hold for no more than ten seconds at a time. Simply lower your knees to the floor, rest for one second then lift again.

Place the dowel along your spine, when performing the exercise. It will give you great feedback on what your spine and trunk are doing.

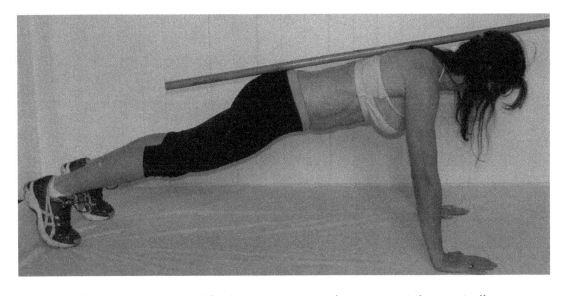

Ensure you do not feel any soreness in your vertebrae at all.

123

Instructions:

Adopt a four-point position as shown. Place your hands and feet on the floor.

Ensure your spine, including your neck, is neutral. Your feet should be hip width apart, and your hands should be directly below your shoulders.

Ensure your core stabilisers are activated to support your vertebrae.

Place the dowel along your vertebrae.

Keep your trunk fixed and lift one hand off the floor. You do not need to lift with a straight arm as for the four-point series, just simply lift one hand off the floor at a time.

Lower that hand down and lift the opposite hand.

Continue to lift alternate hands. Be mindful of the ten second rule. Relax and repeat at each ten second mark or beforehand if you feel anything in your spine.

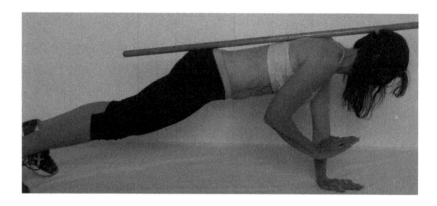

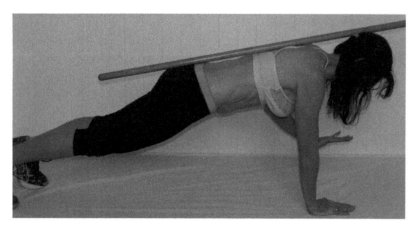

A lot of people will compensate by dropping their head forward, arching in their thoracic spine, dropping their pelvis, and/or lifting their pelvis. If this happens, spinal alignment has been compromised and the potential risk of injury is great.

Correct technique is of the utmost importance at all times.

If you cannot do the exercise without moving your trunk in a compensatory manner, then regress to the previous exercises, until you are stronger.

You want to ensure that your ankles, knees, hips, and shoulders form a straight line that does not deviate at all when you move your limbs.

Repetitions, sets, and exercise duration (hold duration), are all determined by your body. If you feel pain in your vertebrae, you must stop. If you are not doing the exercise correctly, you must stop and regress the exercise.

Do not aim to hold the same contraction for minutes at a time. It is not ideal for your spinal stability. Aim to hold each contraction for ten seconds The factor you can increase is the number of repetitions. Aim for three repetitions initially. Then gradually build up to eight to ten repetitions.

What not to do:

Lifting the pelvis up

Rotating in the trunk or pelvis

Not maintaining spinal stability

Not using your gluteals to extend your leg

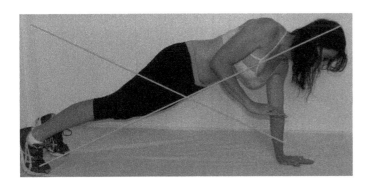 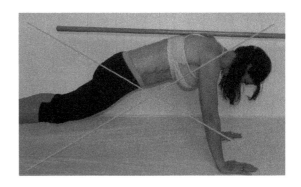

Supine Hip Extension with Single Leg

This exercise is a direct progression from 'Supine Hip Extension Alternate Leg Lift'. Do not progress to this exercise until you can execute that exercise correctly.

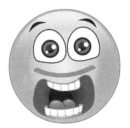

The progression of this exercise is lifting the pelvis up using one leg only. Each time the pelvis is lifted, you need to ensure it raises horizontally, and without dropping or tilting.

The muscles of one leg are doing the lifting, along with ensuring the pelvis remains horizontal. The previous exercise ('Supine Hip Extension Alternate Leg Lift'), required the muscles of both legs to lift the pelvis, then only one to stabilise the pelvis at the top.

Correct muscle activation is important to prevent the lower back muscles from activating and overriding the gluteals.

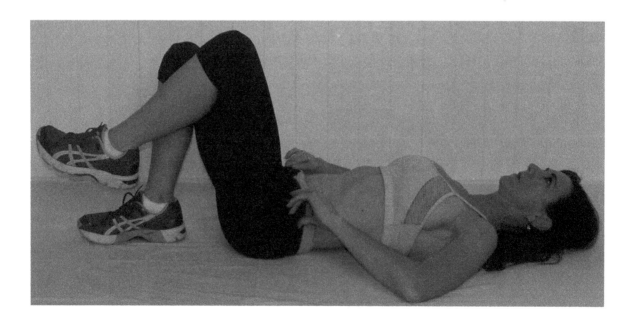

Instructions:

Supine Hip Extension with Single Leg Bent Leg

Ensure your pelvis stays horizontal throughout the entire movement.

Lie on your back. Ensure your spine and pelvis are neutral, that your legs are bent and that your feet are hip width apart.

Activate your pelvic floor and your TrA. Tilt your pelvis backward. (Imagine there is a bowl of water in your pelvis and you are tipping it out on the floor).

This tilting backward of your pelvis places your back muscles on stretch. This makes it hard for them to turn on.

Lift one foot off the floor, and keep that knee bent. Keep your core musculature activated, consciously activate the gluteals of the weight bearing leg. Lift your pelvis off the floor one vertebra at a time.

Once you have reached the top, slowly lower down one vertebra at a time. Return to neutral spine, then work through the activation process again. Make sure the correct muscles are working.

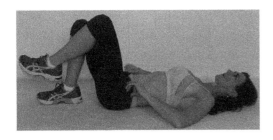

Performing this exercise with your other knee bent is the easiest way. The lever is shorter and therefore, lighter.

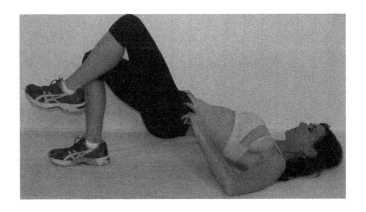

Perform the action for up to ten repetitions, as long as each and every repetition is correct.

Relax down and change legs.

Once you are able to lift your pelvis up, keeping it horizontal with the other leg bent, you can then progress to doing the same action with a straighter leg.

Some readers will find that lifting with one leg is more difficult to keep the pelvis horizontal than lifting with the other. This may or may not be the same leg as with previous exercises.

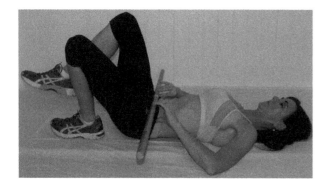

The exercises prescribed here are a combination of static, dynamic, isolation and compound exercises and your body responds differently to each one. This is why there are a number of exercises that are similar with progressions.

It is a good exercise to use the dowel across your pelvis. If there is a slight tilt or drop on one side, having a stick on the bony points will exaggerate the tilt at the end of the stick, so it will be easier to notice.

Remember: the lifting and lowering of the pelvis one vertebra at a time is essential to the success of this exercise. As is the importance of the pelvis staying horizontal.

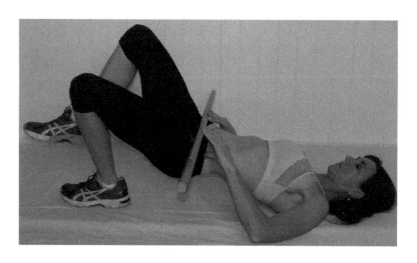

Instructions:

Supine Hip Extension with Single Leg Straight Leg

Lie on your back. Ensure your spine and pelvis are neutral, that your legs are bent and that your feet are hip width apart.

Activate your pelvic floor and TrA. Tilt your pelvis backward. (Imagine there is a bowl of water in your pelvis and you are tipping it out on the floor).

This tilting backward of your pelvis places your back muscles on stretch. This makes it hard for them to turn on.

Lift one foot off the floor and straighten this leg. Keep your core musculature activated, consciously activate the gluteals of the weight bearing leg. Lift your pelvis off the floor one vertebra at a time.

Once you have reached the top, slowly lower down one vertebra at a time. Return to neutral spine, then work through the activation process again, to ensure the correct muscles are working.

Ensure your pelvis stays horizontal throughout the entire movement.

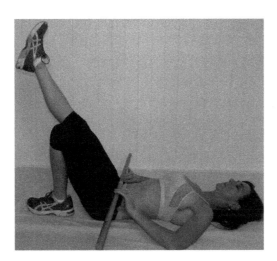

Perform the action for a up to ten repetitions, as long as each and every repetition is correct.

Then relax down and change legs.

129

Some readers will find that lifting with one leg is more difficult to keep the pelvis horizontal than lifting with the other. This may or may not be the same leg as with previous exercises.

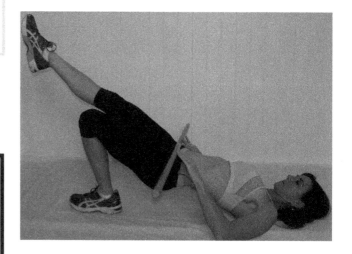

The exercises prescribed here are a combination of static, dynamic, isolation and compound exercises and your body responds differently to each one. This is why there are a number of exercises that are similar with progressions.

Remember: the lifting and lowering of the pelvis one vertebra at a time is essential to the success of this exercise. As is the importance of the pelvis staying horizontal.

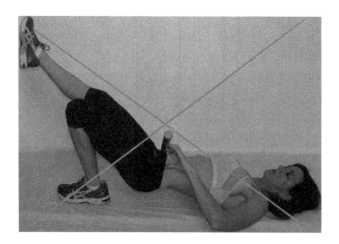

This is a good exercise to use the dowel across your pelvis. If there is a slight tilt or drop on one side, having a stick on the bony points will exaggerate the tilt at the end of the stick, so it will be easier to notice.

Side Plank on Knees

This exercise works a combination of your obliques, your hip abductors, your core musculature and the muscles in your shoulder.

This exercise is a good compound exercise, but one that must be done correctly.

Most of the exercises you have worked through, have been relatively simple in that they are isolation exercises, (using one or two muscle groups to perform an action), or exercises with relatively low loads to lift.

This exercise is a compound exercise, in that more than one muscle group is required to perform the action. It is also more difficult to perform, in that the spine is not supported, except with your trunk musculature. The load lifted can be quite heavy.

This is a progression from a combination of a number of exercises prescribed throughout this book.

Alignment is very commonly poorly executed when people do this exercise.

Be mindful at all times to keep your spine neutral and not allow the weight-bearing shoulder to 'collapse'.

Instructions:

Side Plank on Knees

> Lie on your left side. Ensure your elbow is directly below your shoulder, and you are slightly on your forearm; not the point of your elbow. Your legs should be on top of each other with your knees bent at about ninety degrees, and your pelvis is tucked behind you.

Ensure your spine is neutral. Imagine you have the dowel along your vertebrae and be aware of the need to maintain your three points of contact.

Activate your deep neck flexors, your core musculature, and the obliques and hip abductors of your left side.

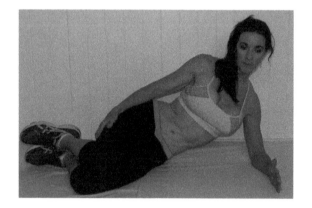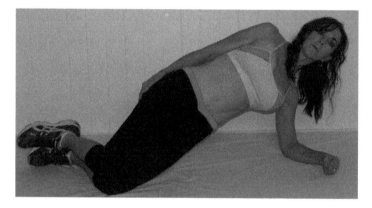

Ensure you have 'set' your shoulder so it does not 'collapse' into itself. Ensure your shoulder blades are drawn down and are sitting flat on your rib cage. Placing the hand of the top arm onto the bottom shoulder and gently pulling that shoulder down can help with correct shoulder positioning.

Aim to bring your pelvis forward, and you should find that your trunk automatically lifts up, so it now forms a straight line from your knees right up through to your nose.

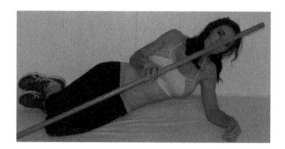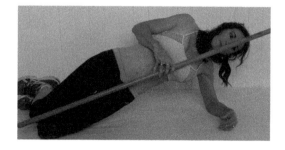

You need to consider alignment in two planes:

From the front; ensure your nose is in line with your sternum and belly button.

From the side; ensure your spine is in the correct position so you would have three points of contact, just as if you had the dowel along your spine.

Hold this position for no more than ten seconds. Your spinal stabilisers are still required to support your vertebrae in this position. Remember: you are working to improve your spinal health, stability, and strength.

As you lower down, ensure you move your pelvis in a backward direction, not just lowering down.

Repeat for a number of repetitions, then change sides.

Once you are able to perform this exercise correctly on your knees, you can progress to doing it on your feet.

What not to do:

Not maintaining spinal alignment

Collapsing in the shoulder

Collapsing in the trunk

Knees starting in line with the trunk

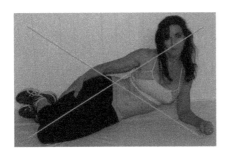 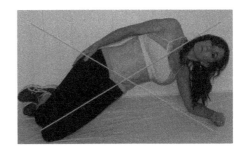

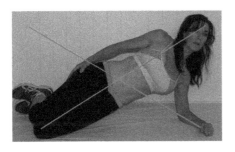 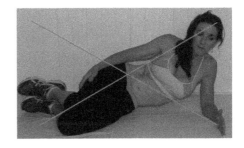

Side Plank on Feet

This exercise works a combination of your obliques, your hip abductors, your core musculature and the muscles in your shoulder.

This exercise is a good compound exercise, but one that must be done correctly.

Most of the exercises you have worked through, have been relatively simple in that they are isolation exercises, (using one or two muscle groups to perform an action), or exercises with relatively low loads to lift.

This exercise is a compound exercise, in that more than one muscle group is required to perform the action. It is also more difficult to perform, in that the spine is not supported, except with your trunk musculature. The load lifted can be quite heavy and is definitely heavier than performing this on your knees.

The load is heavier for the trunk and the shoulder in this exercise compared to 'Side Plank on Knees'. Progress to this exercise when you can perform that exercise properly.

Alignment is very commonly poorly executed when people do this exercise. Use a mirror to check your alignment.

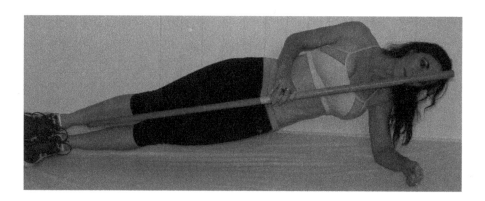

Instructions:

Side Plank On Feet

Lie on your right side. Ensure your elbow is directly below your shoulder, and you are slightly on your forearm; not the point of your elbow.

Your legs should be on top of each other.

Ensure your spine is neutral. Imagine you have the dowel along your vertebrae and be aware of the need to maintain your three points of contact.

Activate your deep neck flexors, your core musculature, and the obliques and hip abductors of your left side.

Ensure you have 'set' your shoulder so it does not 'collapse' into itself. Ensure your shoulder blades are drawn down and are sitting flat on your rib cage. Placing the hand of the top arm onto the bottom shoulder and gently pulling that shoulder down can help with correct shoulder positioning.

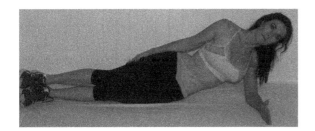

Lift your trunk up so it now forms a straight line from the feet right up through to the nose.

You need to consider alignment in two planes:

From the front; ensure your nose is in line with your sternum and belly button.

From the side; ensure your spine is in the correct position so you would have three points of contact, just as if you had the dowel along your spine.

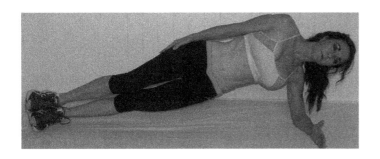

Hold this position for no more than ten seconds. Your spinal stabilisers are still required to support your vertebrae in this position. Remember: you are working to improve your spinal health, stability, and strength.

If you struggle with 'balancing' in this position, you can perform the exercise with your feet in line. (Your top leg will be your front leg). Doing this, you have increased your base of support and you should immediately feel more stable. Aim to progress to performing this with your feet on top of each other.

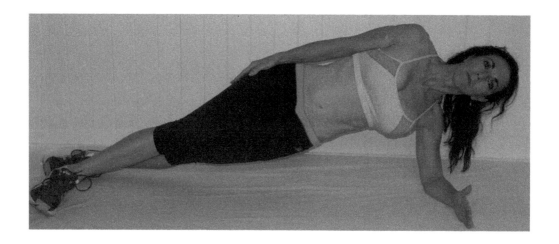

Repeat for a number of repetitions then change sides.

McGill Curl-Up

Dr Stuart McGill is considered a world expert on back health. He recommends to 'preserve the curve', which means spinal alignment should be maintained when performing abdominal exercises.

This exercise has progressions. However, I will only show you the 'McGill Curl-Up'. I hope by now I have stirred a desire in you to further educate yourselves on correct technique with more functional exercises.

My website www.CoreStrengthHQ.com and my You

Tube Channel Core Strength HQ, have a number of exercises detailed with correct technique. I would like to also recommend you look up Dr Stuart McGill for further information on back health and spinal stability.

This exercise integrates a number of anterior chain muscles (muscles in the front of the body). The exercises in this book have taught you how to activate every muscle needed to execute this exercise.

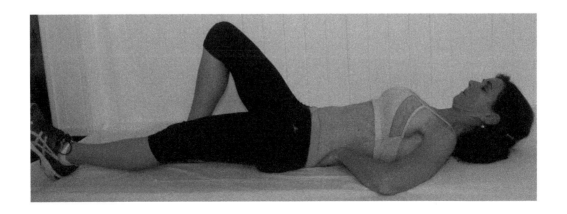

137

Instructions:

McGill Curl-Up

Lie on your back. Bend one knee up, and place that foot on the floor and keep it there.

Clasp your hands together behind your lower back. This should keep your spinal alignment in neutral.

The chest, shoulders, and head lift as one fixed unit. You do not curl or crunch the trunk.

Activate your deep neck flexors and your core stabilisers.

Perform the breathing technique taught with 'Pelvic Floor and Transverse Abdominis Activation', this is essential to do before you lift.

Imagine your head is resting on a set of weight scales, and you want to lift up the 'fixed unit', but you want to imagine your head is still touching the scales and they read zero weight.

Without using your elbows to help you, lift your head and shoulders off the floor.

Lift and hold for up to eight seconds.
Lower the 'fixed unit' down, but keep the trunk activation on. Repeat.
Perform for a number of repetitions, then change the leg that is bent.

Focus on 'stiffness' through the trunk.

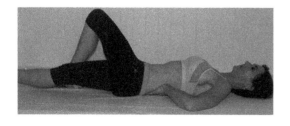
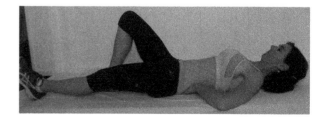

138

Some people will be restricted in their shoulder and unable to place their hand under their lower back. If this is you, then simply grab a towel, and roll it up, place it under your lower back. Roll the towel so far that it supports your spinal curves, and does not exaggerate them.

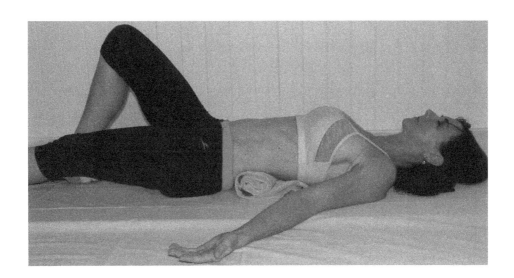

What not to do:

Bend both legs

Straighten both legs

Curl up leading with the head

Crunch in the trunk

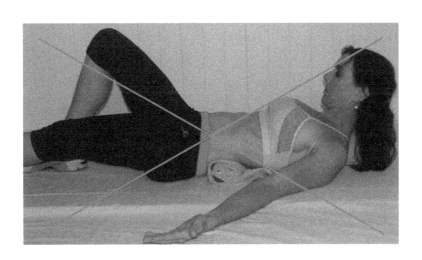

Standing Trunk Rotation with a Band

This exercise is a great way to activate your trunk musculature.

Progress to this exercise once you are able to do all the other exercises shown in this book. If you attempt to do this without awareness of your correct muscle activation, you risk injury to yourself.

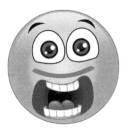

At all times, listen to your body and be very mindful of correct muscle activation and spinal posture.

This exercise can be done with a partner, however, partners can be unpredictable, so at this stage I recommend you use a resistance band.

Start out with a light resistance band and progress to a heavier one, as you are able to.

Instructions:

Standing Trunk Rotation with a Band

Tie a resistance band on something solid. Make sure it is about chest height.

Stand side-on to the resistance band, with it fixed on your left hand side.

Ensure your knees are slightly bent. Keep your feet hip width or slightly wider apart, turn from your trunk to hold the band with both hands.

Ideally, your trunk moves as a fixed unit and your hands remain together, and directly in front of your sternum at all times.

Activate your core musculature and use these muscles to bring your trunk around to the centre. Return to the start position. Ensure you are using your core musculature to control the movement.

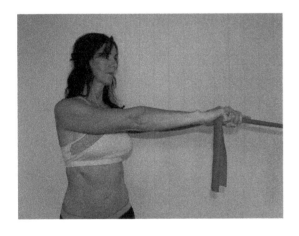

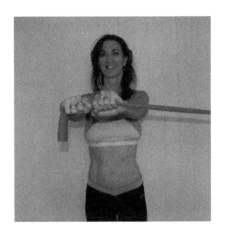

Your core musculature must be on to ensure spinal stability and to help create the movement.

Move in the range that feels comfortable for you, with correct muscle activation.

Perform a set number of repetitions then change sides.

141

Your movement should be slow and controlled.

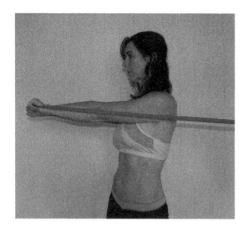

If you are confident and able to perform this action then you can try to turn your trunk the entire way to the right. Ensure your hands stay in line with your sternum.

Note: the thicker the resistance band means the resistance is heavier. The shorter you make the resistance band, also means the resistance is heavier. Find the happy medium of a decent challenge but not too hard that you cannot activate correctly.

At no point should you feel anything in your vertebrae. You may feel the muscles on the sides of your back activating and this is perfectly fine, because you should feel them.

What not to do:

Bent arms

Hands not in line with sternum

Head not following the sternum

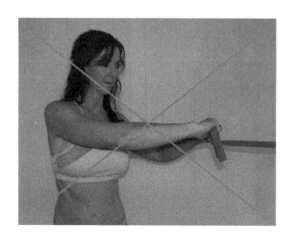 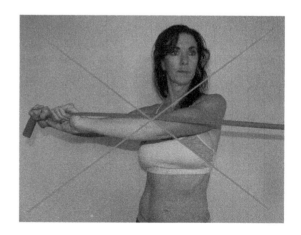

Crab Walk with a Band

This exercise requires core stability and pelvic stability.

Your core musculature must be on to prevent unwanted movement in the trunk while you are moving the legs.

It is important to keep your pelvis horizontal throughout the exercise.

Note: the thicker the resistance band means the resistance is heavier. The shorter you make the resistance band, also means the resistance is heavier. Find the happy medium of a decent challenge but not too hard that you cannot activate correctly.

This is another integration exercise. Your spine is not supported and you will have load on your lower limbs.

Be very mindful of what you are doing at all times.

Ensure you keep your trunk fixed throughout the exercise. Be aware of preventing it from twisting and turning.

143

Crab Walk with a Band

Tie a resistance band in a loop. The smaller the loop, the heavier the resistance will be.

You want to feel resistance throughout the majority of the step, not just at the end range.

You will need to find the happy medium of a decent challenge with resistance throughout the movement, without it being too hard. And not too soft that you can only feel the resistance at the end of the step.

> Stand in the loop and place the band on your ankles.

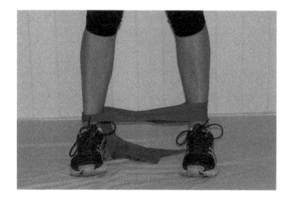

> Keep your spine and neck neutral. Activate your core musculature.

Take a big step sideways to the right. Ensure your pelvis stays horizontal, and that your trunk does not twist.

> Bring the left leg to the lead (right) leg, with control. Step again to the right and bring the left leg to the right leg.

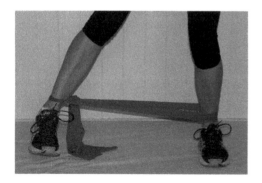

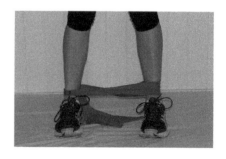

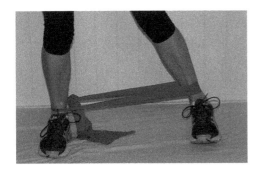 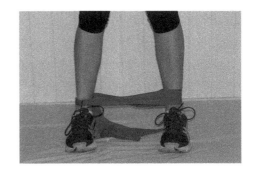

Continue to take a number of steps to the right. Then step to the left. Bring the right leg to the left with control. Continue until you have repeated the same number of repetitions in each direction.

This exercise can be progressed to stepping at a forty five degree angle. Always be very mindful of your trunk and pelvis staying fixed.

Remember that your sets and repetitions are determined by your technique.

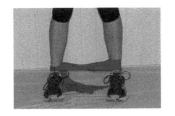 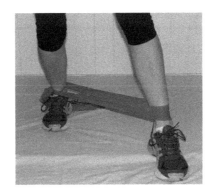 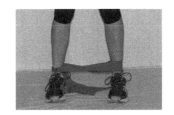

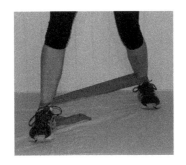

Stand in the loop and place the band on your ankles. Step forward at a forty five degree angle with your left leg.

Bring your right leg in to the start position.

Step forward at a forty five degree angle with your right leg.

Continue stepping forward for a number of steps.

Once you have control you can progress to the same action but in reverse. Ensure you use your gluteals to extend your leg back.

At all times keep your trunk fixed.

The Wind-Up

You have done really well to get to here.

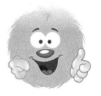

I am assuming you have gradually worked through this book, as recommended.

This may have taken some time, depending on what stage you were at when you started reading this book.

If you have reached here, it should mean, you are feeling stronger, more mobile, and more able to perform activities of daily life. You should be feeling less pain in your back, and more confident to do things you have not been able to do in the past, due to pain restrictions.

It is important you have learned to be mindful of correct muscle activation with movements. Eventually, your neuromuscular system will know how to activate your core musculature without you having to consciously think about it. If your core musculature is functioning correctly, it should activate thirty to fifty milli-seconds before you move a limb.

However, I would recommend when you are lifting anything heavy, you stop, think, ensure you have activated the right muscles, then lift.

There will be exercises and stretches in this book that you found very beneficial. At any time you can return to these activities and perform them. It is not necessarily a regression in your program. It is a necessity to 'remind' your neuromuscular system what it needs to do. It is also good to re-visit these exercises at times when performing your usual exercise program.

Rotations are a fantastic stretch to do whenever your back feels tight. These can be done before you do any exercise.

Remember the purpose of a stretch is to relax tight muscles and, to elongate a muscle if you so desire. The stretches in this book are designed to help deactivate, or turn off, facilitated muscles. To gain the most benefit from these stretches, perform them before your exercise program and throughout your workout, especially when you notice the facilitated muscles are starting to override the other muscles again.

I have quite often had clients stretch at the outset, then perform a number of repetitions. As soon as it is noticed the facilitated muscle is again activated and preventing the other muscles from doing their job properly, I have them stretch the 'problem muscle/s' again, then exercise again. This stop-to-stretch activity may occur as many times as is necessary in one workout. It really depends on how responsive the muscles are.

Prehabilitation - the prevention of injury. It is important to keep on top of your core strength and stability. You have come so far, don't lose what you have gained.

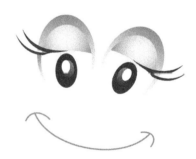

The intention of this book is to help you equip yourself with the knowledge of what actions certain muscles perform.

The descriptions of the muscles including diagrams, are very basic. It is hoped I have raised curiosity in you to find out more about our fascinating bodies and how they work.

Index

A

Achilles 148

alignment 15, 56, 59, 61-63, 65, 70, 86, 99-101, 104, 120, 123, 125, 131, 133-135, 137-138, 148

B

balance 41, vi, 54, 148-151

balance challenges 148

before you start 148

benefits of a regular exercise program 148

blood pressure 10, 148

Bodyblade 148

C

calf stretch 148

cardiovascular exercises 148

centre of gravity 148

chin retraction 148

D

duraDisc 148, 150-151

dynamic lunge 100, 148

E

exercises 6 148

F

feet on duraDisc 148

finding neutral spine/neutral pelvis 148

foam balance beam 148-151